▶ The Attention Deficit Disorder in Adults Workbook

Dr. Lynn Weiss

Taylor Publishing Company

Dallas, Texas

Also by Lynn Weiss

————————————

Attention Deficit Disorder in Adults

Power Lines (with Lora Cain)

I Wasn't Finished with Life (with Dorothy and Judy Thatch)

Freedom To Grow (with Angie Rose)

Emotionally Yours

Copyright © 1994 Lynn Weiss

All rights reserved.

Published by Taylor Publishing Company
1550 West Mockingbird Lane
Dallas, Texas 75235
(800) 677-2800 x319

Designed by Hespenheide Design

Printed in the United States of America
10   9   8   7   6   5   4

Contents

Chapter 1 Introduction

Chapter 2 Assessment

Chapter 3 Coping with Your ADD

Chapter 4 Essential Skills

Chapter 5   Living Up to Your Potential

Chapter 6   Continuing Your Education

Index

Acknowledgments

This workbook is dedicated to people who have ADD. As each of you has contacted me in person, by phone, and in writing, another bit of the ADD story has been told. You've let me know what you need, and part of my response is contained in these pages. Together we constructed this book.

I thank you for your openness and heartfelt sensitivity as you have shared your special way of experiencing the world, the ADD way. I applaud your drive and courage to become powerful, effective members of our society. I reinforce the esteem that builds in each of you. May your potential be your companion.

Thanks to family and friends who support the ADD interest.

I wish to express gratitude to my professional companions who work in the trenches to unearth wonderful new discoveries about ADD; lauding the assets and taming the challenges.

A major vote of thanks to Mary Kelly, who continues to teach me to write and think at a higher level than I knew was possible and who believes in me. Thanks to Holly McGuire, who steered me through the publication process, and to all the people at Taylor Publishing Company for their support in bringing ADD to the attention of the public.

And finally, thank you to the members of my spiritual family, who surround me with love, understanding, and a good swift boot in the backside when needed!

Chapter 1
Introduction

▶ ## Note to Reader

Dear Reader,

My experience with attention deficit disorder in adults began when my son, diagnosed with ADD as a child, went through puberty with his ADD intact. Together we discovered many things that helped him make the transition to adulthood with minimum impairment.

Thanks to the opportunity to work with many teens and adults who have ADD, I learned first hand from the people who live and cope with the condition every day. Along with the help of their spouses and friends, I received the best training available. In the late 1980s little was written about ADD, so the mandate to put on paper what I discovered about ADD was handed to me.

Since the 1991 publication of *Attention Deficit Disorder in Adults,* I have been privileged to meet and work with hundreds of people whose lives have been touched by ADD. Evaluations uncovered many previously undiagnosed individuals. I then discovered a great need for training and education guidance to cope with ADD.

This workbook is the result. It includes descriptions, worksheets, and motivational material to support you as you, too, learn to cope with ADD. As the people in my training and education groups in Dallas, Texas, have come to find out, you deserve the same opportunity to live up to your potential as anyone without ADD has. No matter what your circumstances, you are a valuable person. Remember that.

People who have been assessed with ADD have joined in helping to educate all of us. They are wanting to give back. As a result a video has been produced, *Adult Attention Deficit*

1

Disorder (WW Productions, 1993). It demonstrates the sensitivity that characterizes all people with ADD. Through their sharing they make all of us more aware of what ADD is about. Similarly, your sensitivity makes you more creative and more empathetic. Both attributes are much needed in today's society as we strive to meet the challenges of the twenty-first century. Your ability to see the world in new ways will enable you to be on the cutting edge of much-needed developments.

You *are* special. Don't for one minute think that you are less valuable than the next guy. With a little guidance, you will be able to harness the assets you have and enjoy the results of your successes. I believe in you. Begin now to believe in yourself.

Affectionately and sincerely,

Dr. Lynn Weiss

▶ Purpose

Reading about ADD is one thing. Coping with your ADD is quite another. The purpose of this workbook is to help you be able to do something about it.

My experience has shown me that people with ADD are eager to make changes.

As you use this book, you can expect to

▷ recognize ADD symptoms in yourself.
▷ find ways to cope with your ADD.
▷ feel good about yourself.
▷ be able to work to your potential.
▷ get in control of your life.

You can get in control of your life by

▷ reducing the effects of your past.
▷ handling your feelings.
▷ getting organized.
▷ achieving the goals you set.
▷ developing interpersonal skills.
▷ learning to relax.
▷ learning to use resources.

In this step-by-step guide, you will discover a proven method of bringing order and happiness to your life. You will improve yourself and become more effective in your life.

▶ How to Use This Book

This book is divided into sections so that you can easily find areas to work on that interest you. Start wherever you want. You do not need to use the Workbook in any special order. Feel free to be creative in your approach.

Due to the fact that most people with ADD do better with a structure, you may want to simply start at the beginning and work straight through the book, skipping items that are not a problem for you.

You do not have to do all of the exercises in the book. You can do as many or as few as you want.

No one knows as well as you do what is bothering you, causing trouble in your life, or in need of attention. It's up to you whether you choose to work on a tough area or begin with something small and easier to deal with.

If at any time you feel anxious while using the materials, it is all right to set them aside. You may be onto something that needs attention in your life, and working with a counselor could be in order.

Chapter 2

Assessment

▶ Do I Have ADD or Not?

Determining whether you have attention deficit disorder involves two steps.

▷ **Step 1:** You screen yourself for the disorder.
▷ **Step 2:** If it seems likely that you do have it, you next need to consult a professional who works with ADD in adults.
  A. You will then find out for sure if you have ADD.
  B. You will discover whether other conditions are present.
  C. You may discover you don't have ADD but you have something else.

Here's a checklist that you can use to determine whether or not you probably have ADD. It will help you decide if you want to be formally assessed. If you do not show many of the signs of ADD here, you will need to look for other causes for your difficulties. Consult with a counselor or psychotherapist.

Now, begin the assessment.

A SELF-ASSESSMENT

As a child,
did you have problems paying attention when you were in school?

_____ yes _____ no

was it hard for you to concentrate?

_____ yes _____ no

were you always on the go?

_____ yes _____ no

did you talk a lot even when you were trying to be quiet?

_____ yes _____ no

was it difficult for you to sit still or stay in your seat?

_____ yes _____ no

Now that you are a grown-up,
do you have problems paying attention at work?

_____ yes _____ no

is it hard for you to concentrate?

_____ yes _____ no

are you always on the go?

_____ yes _____ no

do you still talk a lot, even interrupting sometimes?

_____ yes _____ no

is it hard for you to sit still or stay in your seat during meetings?

_____ yes _____ no

If you answered "yes" to most of these questions, you can begin to suspect that you may have ADD.
  ▷ ADD is always present from childhood; if you didn't experience any of these symptoms in childhood, you don't have ADD.
  ▷ It is not something that begins later in life.
  ▷ You don't just begin to have concentration problems because of ADD when you are eleven or twenty-three or forty-five.

If you do not seem to have ADD, you need to know that your problems are real, but the cause is not ADD.

If you answered "no" to most of them, especially the first set, you do not have ADD. Two of the following five categories must be present for a diagnosis of ADD to be warranted.

1. IMPULSIVITY

As a child,
did you act impulsively a lot of the time?

_____ yes   _____ no

was it hard or impossible for you to wait your turn?

_____ yes   _____ no

As a grown-up,
do you often do things without thinking?

_____ yes   _____ no

do you find yourself wishing you had spent more time planning things?

_____ yes   _____ no

2. LOW STRESS TOLERANCE AND OVERREACTIONS

As a child,
did you make a big deal out of little things?

_____ yes   _____ no

were you often accused of overreacting?

_____ yes   _____ no

As a grown-up,
do you fly off the handle easily?

_____ yes   _____ no

does life seem overly stressful much of the time?

_____ yes   _____ no

7

3. POOR ORGANIZATION AND TASK COMPLETION

As a child,
was it hard for you to finish things?

_____ yes _____ no

did you find it was hard to get or stay organized?

_____ yes _____ no

As a grown-up,
do you have difficulty finishing things?

_____ yes _____ no

are you often confused or do you have trouble finding things?

_____ yes _____ no

4. EXTREME MOOD SWINGS

As a child,
was it easy for others to get you overly excited or upset?

_____ yes _____ no

did you feel down whenever something bad happened around you?

_____ yes _____ no

As a grown-up,
do your moods depend on what happens to you during a day?

_____ yes _____ no

does your mood change because of what someone else does or says?

_____ yes _____ no

5. SHORT, EXCESSIVE TEMPER

As a child,
were you considered a hothead?

_____ yes   _____ no

did you get very upset easily?

_____ yes   _____ no

As a grown-up,
do you get angry easily?

_____ yes   _____ no

does your temper get out of control?

_____ yes   _____ no

In order to be diagnosed with ADD, you must have "yes" responses in at least two of the five child sections.

Add up the "yes" responses you have as a grown-up. If you have fewer "yes" responses as an adult than as a child, you have been successfully working on overcoming the effects of ADD.

If your adult "yes" responses are greater than your "yes" responses as a child, your problems are probably caused by something other than ADD. Remember, the symptoms **must** be present in childhood to be considered ADD.

If you have many of the attributes characteristic of someone with ADD, get a formal evaluation. This will open many doors for you to get help with your condition. If it turns out that you do not have ADD, ask the person doing the testing to show you how to get help for your particular problem.

To begin working with your ADD, continue.

Chapter 3
Coping with Your ADD

▶ Getting Ready to Go to Work

With a little preparation, you increase the probability that you will succeed in learning to cope effectively with your ADD. It will be easier if you have a proper mind-set, self-talk, and the following tips.

Your mind set is very important.

▷ To work effectively on your ADD, you must decide that you want to do it.
▷ You must make a commitment to do the best you can.
▷ You need to persevere even when you don't feel like it. Take a short rest, then return to working on your ADD.
▷ You must realize that you are worthwhile and are made of the stuff that winners are made of.

Use positive self-talk. Tell yourself:

"I want to work on my ADD."
"I choose to do the best I can."
"Even if I don't feel like it, I'll go back to my work on my ADD after a rest."
"I am worthwhile."
"I am a winner."

Put signs up that remind you of these points.
Develop a buddy system.
Ask a friend to help with your ADD.
If you are in a support group, choose someone to help you.
Choose a relative to work with you on your program.
You may return the favor directly by being a buddy to someone else.

11

Consult with a counselor.

> ▷ Find someone who is interested in ADD and in you.
> ▷ Learn from the person.
> ▷ Share your feelings with the counselor.
> ▷ Practice your new skills on the person.

▶ The Formal Evaluation

You must be assessed to see whether you have ADD.

> ▷ Finding a professional to do the assessment:
> Professionals who work in the field of ADD often have a special interest in the subject and will write or talk about ADD.
>> Look in books.
>> Listen to talks.
>> Go to lectures.
>> Read articles.
>> Contact your Mental Health Association.
>> Ask your doctor or school personnel.
>> Check with a university.
>> Look for a support group for children with ADD.
>> Look for a support group for adults with ADD.
>>> (See the appendix of *Attention Deficit Disorder in Adults,* Taylor Publishing Company, 1991.)
>> Subscribe to a newsletter about ADD in adults.
> ▷ Professionals who may assess ADD include

Psychologists	Counselors
Psychiatrists	Social Workers
Educational Diagnosticians	Pediatricians
Adolescent Physicians	Educators
Graduate students affiliated with a university clinic or research project	

> ▷ Call for an appointment. (Ask about what experience he or she has had with adult ADD, fees, what you get for your money, and the time involved.) Be sure you will get a written report with recommendations for treatment. You will need to sign a release so your report may be shared with other professionals. This is necessary if you seek medication or special services.

After you have been officially diagnosed, you need a plan of attack to deal with your ADD. This workbook offers you a practical approach to coping with your condition. You may choose to work through this book on your own, with a therapist or tutor, or within an ADD support group.

▶ Overview of Program

In general, your program of dealing with ADD will include the following steps.

▷ Follow up on the recommendations you were given when you were diagnosed.

▷ Seek group or individual counseling. I've found short-term training in a group is excellent to learn coping skills.

First, heal old, hurt feelings.
Second, gain control of your impulses and temper.
Then, rework your values.
Next, tackle organizational skills, interpersonal relations, and job-related issues.
All of this will take time, but you're worth it.

▷ Work in depth on remaining weak areas using this workbook either by yourself or with a counselor.

▷ You will begin to think of yourself differently—as someone with ADD. This is a big change in your identity. Work on updating your view of yourself, taking your ADD into account.

▷ Begin to plan lifestyle changes that reflect the new you.

▷ Join a support group for ADD in your local area or consider starting one.

You may be able to cut counseling back to monthly check-ins to be sure you are on track. If you are working with the workbook on your own, schedule monthly checkups to keep track of your progress. Later you can do this quarterly.

▶ Commitment

Whether or not you get counseling or join a support group, the only person who can get control of your ADD is you. Therefore, you will need to make a real commitment to this process. I'm asking you to complete and sign the following commitment pledge.

I ask you to make a commitment to do the best you can to remedy the difficulties that result from your having ADD. You do not need to be perfect—just do your best!

I commit to do my best to help myself.

_____   _____

Name   Date

Despite your best intentions, you will sometimes fall short of goals and lapse in progress. It is only human.

What can you do if you fall off the ADD track? It's very simple. **Get back on track.**

I commit to get back on track if I fall off.

_____   _____

Name   Date

▶ Understanding Grief

Grief is a natural response to losing someone or something. Change, even positive change, creates feelings of loss and, therefore, grief.

You are likely to grieve when

▷ You lose **something** that was important to you, such as
1. a job
2. a pet
3. a hobby or pastime
4. a way of life
5. your health
6. a possession or keepsake
7. income
8. time
9. an expectation

▷ You lose **someone** (through death, divorce, moving, or voluntary or involuntary separation) whom you:
1. have cared about
2. are or have been committed to
3. lived with
4. admired
5. loved
6. were related to

▶ Grief and ADD

As a person with ADD, you are especially likely to grieve when

▷ you lose something you desire, such as
1. a dream
2. the ability to reach your potential

▷ or when you feel cheated out of
1. the opportunity to achieve what you want
2. the opportunity to live out normal stages of development
3. a part of your youth
4. the ability to produce effectively
5. the ability to achieve success or know why you haven't

List here some things you have lost directly because of your ADD.

_____

_____

_____

Did you know that:

▷ most people with ADD feel the same way you do.

▷ it's okay to grieve your losses. They are real. You don't have to feel bad about these losses forever.

▷ you can do something about it.

People with ADD suffer all kinds of losses because of their condition. Some are listed here.

1. Your ADD may have prevented you from getting as far in your education as you wanted and know you are capable of.

2. Your ADD may have interfered with opportunities to pursue sports, a musical instrument, or some other special interest.

3. Maybe your ADD made high school so unpleasant for you that you dropped out and took a minimum-wage job.

4. Your ADD might be keeping you from doing your best at work. Maybe you can't ever get your paperwork done or your sales reports turned in.

5. Maybe you have not gotten promotions or landed accounts or even gotten jobs because of your ADD.

6. Perhaps your temper may have cost you relationships that matter to you.

▶ Stages of Grief

Let's begin to work on grieving those losses. To understand how to heal grief, here is what you must know.

▷ Healing is a process.

▷ Healing involves **five stages.**

STAGE ONE: DENIAL

Denial is characterized by a failure to perceive the experience or realize your feelings about the loss you suffered.

People in denial say, "I can't understand what's wrong with me." You may experience confusion or a sense of unreality about what's wrong with you.

You may cover your feelings with some addiction, such as drugs, alcohol, work, busy-ness, excitement, new projects, running, video games, computer projects, food, sex, or religion. The list goes on and on.

STAGE TWO: ANGER

Anger is characterized by blaming others for your problems or blowing up easily to cover your feelings of vulnerability.

Anger is a cover-up emotion. Visualize a shield held in front of you that protects your vulnerable body from attack. That's what anger does.

Angry people say things like, "It was the school's fault," or, "It's not fair," or, "I'm not dumb," or "I don't care about making good grades."

You may blame your lack of success on others. You may feel resentful about your troubles and lash out on the highway by shouting at other drivers.

Or you may take it out on your child because he has the same problems you did in school. His lack of success reminds you of your pain.

You may criticize your spouse for not doing the housework well enough, displacing your anger on her.

STAGE THREE: BARGAINING/GUILT

This stage of the grief process gives you the illusion that there is something you can do about your situation. People in this stage say things like, "If only you'll let me get a good review at work, God, I'll promise to work harder next quarter," or "It's all my fault I failed. I'm just dumb and lazy."

If you are bargaining, you may feel that you can cut a deal with someone or something in the future in exchange for being rescued now.

If you feel guilty, you are clinging to the belief that *you* can control the outcome.

STAGE FOUR: DEPRESSION

Depression is the fourth step in the grief process. In this stage, you let yourself feel the loss. Though a normal part of grieving, it can easily pull you down so you can't think clearly. Sometimes it's helpful to think that depression is anger turned in toward yourself. At any rate, you are truly feeling the sadness of the loss at this point and are nearing the end of the grief process.

Depressed people say things like, "I'm just no good," or I'll never be able to do any better. What's the use?"

You may make critical remarks about yourself. You may lose sleep or your appetite, or you may eat more.

Occasionally you may become so discouraged and hopeless that you think of injuring yourself. The depression is creating these feelings. You must get counseling help immediately. Often medication for depression is quite helpful.

There's no need to suffer—it won't help you overcome your grief.

STAGE FIVE: ACCEPTANCE

By this final stage, you will be willing and able to accept your loss and go on with your life. Only at this point is it possible to forgive yourself and others, realizing that everyone involved did the best they could—you included.

People in the acceptance stage say things like, "I am an okay person even though I have ADD," and "Though my teacher (or parent) was wrong, I realize she didn't know any better. I survived and I can now forgive her."

You may experience clarity and insight about your situation.

You may feel renewed hopefulness that, despite your ADD, you can reach some of your dreams.

You may be able to forgive those who hurt you out of ignorance.

Do not force yourself into the forgiveness process. It will happen automatically when the other four stages are completed.

And do not let others, however well-meaning, tell you, "You should forgive them" or "That was years ago" or "Just go on with your life." You have the right to grieve fully the losses ADD has caused in your life. Moreover, only you know what those losses are or how severe each one is.

Now, begin to grieve.

▶ Grieving Your Own ADD

The first step in your grief process is to find out which stage or stages of grief you are currently experiencing. If, for example, you are detached, you are likely to be in the stage of denial. Feeling angry indicates you are in the anger stage. Trying to cut a bargain means you are in stage three and if you are feeling depressed, you are in stage four.

Go back to page 15, where you listed all of the losses you have experienced due to your ADD. Try to determine where you are in the grief process for each.

If you are unsure, breathe slowly, inhaling fully and completely, hold your breath to the count of three, and exhale completely. Repeat several times. Then ask yourself what you are feeling about having ADD.

If you are still unsure, take some time over the next few weeks (this may even take months) to reflect on your losses.

This grieving process is an extremely important part of moving on and deserves all the time it takes.

Let yourself grieve because you have ADD and have lost some of your potential. Take as long as you want.

The next exercise will help facilitate the grief process.

▶ The Worst Year of Your Childhood

What was the most difficult year of your childhood? Get a mental picture in your mind of the age you are thinking about. "I am _____ years old." You may want to get out an old photo of yourself at that age. Even if you feel that all your childhood years were difficult, choose one that was representative.

Describe in detail.

What was going on that year?_____

_____

_____

_____

What did you feel then?_____

_____

_____

_____

What do you feel **now,** as you remember those events?_____

_____

_____

_____

If thinking about your youth makes you feel upset, feel free to put this down for a while and do something different. On the other hand, you may want to get it over with and would rather go forward.

▶ A Letter to Your Child

Write a letter to that child (adolescent) part of you to make him or her feel better. Try talking to that child. If you feel shame or guilt, feelings of helplessness or hopelessness, anger, or worthlessness, or if you feel overwhelmed when you think about him or her, proceed to "Obstacles to Grief" below. Then, return here when you are able.

In your letter, include

1. A statement about getting in touch with that part of yourself. You might say something like, "I'm so glad I found you again and remembered what it felt like to grow up with ADD."
2. A statement of acceptance of the way the child tried to succeed despite the ADD. You might say something like, "I know you did the best you could at the time."
3. A statement giving the child permission to feel angry about what happened. You could say, "It's okay to feel angry about what happened." Feel free to list the people who hurt the child, even if it was out of ignorance. Or, you might say, "I know how angry you feel about your third-grade teacher making you miss recess because you hadn't finished your work."
4. Supportive comments. "I love you. You are very special to me. I'm proud of what you've been able to do, even though you've had the handicap of ADD."
5. Recognition of the child's right to live in a happy manner. You might say, "You deserve to feel happy, and I'm going to see that you get the opportunities."
6. Commitment to remain aware of the child within. Tell your child, "I'll be with you from here on out."

Feel free to add anything you want to the letter. Be sure to put it in your own words. Make it as long or short as you want.

You may become very touched as you do this. That's because you are likely to grieve for the child within you. It's natural to cry.

▶ Obstacles to Grief

Sometimes it's difficult to undergo the grief process because emotional blocks interfere. Typical sources of difficulty are listed here. See which ones fit you.

What gets in the way of being kind to your inner child?

Shame: A deep, painful feeling that something is very wrong with the core of you. Shame makes all of you feel awful.

You must realize that shame is learned from those around you. It is never present nor does it ever develop because there is really something wrong with you. Your ADD is nothing to feel shame about. Someone taught you that it is very shameful to be or act a certain way.

If you feel ashamed of your ADD, tell yourself, "I have nothing to feel shame about."

Write it: _____

_____

You may have to repeat this to yourself a number of times over the next few weeks.

Guilt: Also learned, it makes you feel as if you have responsibility for your ADD and "should" have been able to do things despite it. Feelings of guilt give you the illusion that you could control your ADD, if you tried harder.

You must realize that guilt is learned from people who don't understand the way ADD works. They may have expected you to control your ADD or work at 110% all the time. You *do* have the responsibility to learn how to work with your ADD and do all you can to get it under control. But you are *not* responsible for having ADD. You will often need to accommodate your ADD, making adjustments in your environment so you can be successful.

Tell yourself, "I do not need to feel guilty for having ADD."

Write it: _____

_____

Tell yourself, "I have responsibility for learning to live successfully with my ADD, and I can do it.

Write it: _____

_____

_____

Helplessness: A deep feeling of powerlessness to get your needs met.

Hopelessness: A feeling of desperation. Neither you nor anyone else can do anything to help your situation.

You must realize that helplessness and hopelessness are only feelings that you learned because you did not know what to do about having ADD. Information and learning can provide you with the power to overcome these feelings.

Tell yourself, "I can learn what to do to overcome feelings of helplessness and hopelessness I may have."

Write it: _____

_____

Repeat again and again "I am powerful."

Write it: _____

_____

Anger: An emotion toward someone or something that seems threatening. It is expressed verbally or physically. Its job is to protect us. It simply requires limits to keep it under control.

You must realize that anger is a cover-up emotion that is trying to protect you from your feeling of vulnerability. You deserve to be protected but can find other ways to do it. Anger serves a purpose. It is present to try to help you cope with feelings that threaten your well-being. It's a natural response. It is important to separate the feelings of anger from the behavior you use to express the anger.

Say, "I choose to protect my feelings of vulnerability."

Write it: _____

_____

Say, "I can express my feelings of anger verbally."

Write it: _____

_____

Say, "I can and I choose to control my expression of anger, releasing it in safe, responsible ways."

Write it: _____

_____

Worthlessness: A feeling of having no value. It is a response to feeling inadequate to deal with a situation. It is the sense that you do not deserve success or happiness.

You must realize that feelings of worthlessness are often the outgrowth of depression. They are inaccurate because no one is worthless or less valuable than anyone else.

Tell yourself, "I am a valuable person."

Write it: _____

_____

Say, "I deserve to feel happy and successful."

Write it: _____

_____

Overwhelmed: Feeling overwhelmed is the result of having too many expectations or requirements of yourself without having time to respond. It means you have not been able to set limits on the amount of input you're subjected to.

You must realize that feeling overwhelmed is a natural reaction to overload. Generally it simply requires time to sort out and order whatever is being requested of you. It is up to you to set the limits on the amount of input you are expected to process.

Say, "I can sort through what I need to, at my own pace."

Write it: _____

_____

Say, "I am able to set priorities on the work I do."

Write it: _____

_____

Say, "I can set limits on the amount of input I'm willing to accept at any one time."

Write it: _____

_____

▶ Expressing Grief

It is important to express your grief in whatever way is comfortable for you. There is no **right** way to grieve. People do it differently. Consider using any of the following:

CRYING

Crying is one way. Get the tissues out and give yourself permission to cry. You may want to go away alone for a half day to do this. Or you may prefer to be with someone. Some people prefer to cry in the shower.

If you feel like you want to cry but can't get the tears started, you can rent a sad movie or read a sad book that gets the tears flowing.

HOWLING

Walking in the country and howling or calling to the moon is another way to grieve. This may include kicking a stone down the road, speaking out loud, or repetitively doing an activity like pitching acorns over a cliff. You are symbolically throwing your grief away.

REPETITIVE WORK

Some people prefer to do a repetitive building project such as laying a brick path or pruning a hedge. The action helps move the grief energy through your feelings. You can assist the process by seeing the grief soak into the ground or be discharged into the mortar.

CREATIVE EXPRESSION OF GRIEF

Storytelling, writing, painting, or making music is another way to release emotion.

TALKING IT OUT

Seeking out another person to talk with about your feelings is another way to release grief. It's important to find someone who

is comfortable around feelings
is a good listener
does not tell you what to do or how to do
does not rush you
will keep what you tell him or her confidential

Decide which of the ways you want to grieve. Record your choices below. You may choose one or many ways. You may choose ways that are not listed here.

I choose to grieve by:

_____

_____

and _____

_____

and _____

_____

As you complete your grieving, you will have more emotional energy to work with your ADD. And you will be ready for the next step, forgiving yourself.

I believe (feel) I've completed my grieving, at least for now.

_____
Date and initial

I'm ready to move on to the forgiveness stage.

_____
Initial

▶ Personal Forgiveness

After you have finished grieving, it's time to take one more step. Forgive yourself for all the troubles you've had in relation to ADD. You did the best you knew how at the time. Now you simply know more.

Forgiveness is the pot of gold at the end of the rainbow. However, do not try to force this step. Grieve as long as you need to.

When you are ready, proceed with forgiving yourself.

Right now, right here, I ask you to forgive yourself for any and all inadequacies from which you have suffered.

Today, _____,
                                        date

I, _____,
                                name

forgive myself for any and all inadequacies from which I have suffered in relation to my ADD.

_____
                    signature

Today, _____,
                              date

I, _____,
                        name

forgive myself for any and all inadequacies from which I have suffered in relation to my ADD.

_____
                  signature

Cut out this card and carry it with you.

▶ Pledge of Responsibility

In addition to forgiving yourself, you now will benefit from making a commitment to live responsibly from here on out with your ADD.

Consider the following commitments. They will help you live responsibly.

Taking full responsibility from this day forth for my actions and my thoughts, I
   commit to be the kind of person I admire.
I will ask for help if I don't know what to do next. I will treat myself well in
   thought, word, and deed.
I commit to live a responsible life.

Today, _____,
                                      date

I, _____,
                                   name

commit to live a responsible life, asking for help when I need it and treating
myself well in thought, word, and deed.

_____
                          signature

Tape the large-size pledge in a permanent place (such as your mirror or refrigerator). Cut out the small pledge and carry it with you.

Today, _____,
                   date

I, _____,
                 name

commit to live a responsible life, asking for help
when I need it and treating myself well in
thought, word, and deed.

_____
               signature

Cut out this card and carry it with you.

27

▶ Handling Feelings

Feelings underlie your state of mind and your behavior. They express the needs that you have and let you know when you are getting off track in the fulfillment of them. By learning to recognize and handle your feelings, you will take a big step toward getting attention deficit disorder under control.

Common feelings that you are likely to experience are

_____ Happy	_____ Carefree	_____ Motivated
_____ Curious	_____ Confident	_____ Relaxed
_____ Angry	_____ Fearful	_____ Enraged
_____ Anxious	_____ Nervous	_____ Panicky
_____ Sad	_____ Compulsive	_____ Depressed
_____ Ashamed	_____ Resentful	_____ Guilty
_____ Bored	_____ Excited	
_____ Other _____	_____ Other _____	

Look at the preceding list.

Put a 1 by the feelings you have a lot of the time.
Put a 2 by the feelings you have sometimes.
Put a 3 by the feelings you rarely have.

Next,

Put a + by the ones you like.
Put a – by the ones you want to change.

You get to keep any feeling you like. Put a star by those.

REALIZE

▷ Feelings are always valid.
▷ You only need to change the way in which a feeling is expressed.
▷ Feelings serve a purpose. They are a response to something that has or has not happened.
▷ Your job is to find another way to act on your feelings so that the cost to you or others is reduced.

To begin, it is helpful to consider the following:

Which feelings are a part of normal life?
Which need to be worked with so you can live a normal life?

29

Go back to the list of feelings. Select the first feeling marked with a 3 that you want to change.

Write it here. _____

To determine whether what you are feeling is normal, ask yourself the following:

Am I feeling similar to what other people around me
    feel in the same situation?
Am I told that I am overreacting?
Do people get upset with me when I express my feelings?

Sometimes it is necessary to ask someone you trust whether what you are feeling is normal or not. If you are unsure after you've checked with healthy friends or a mentor, ask a counselor to help you.

Remember: As you learned earlier, feelings that are a part of grief (anger, guilt, depression) are perfectly normal. However, if the same feelings last more than a couple of years after the loss, they are no longer normal, though they are understandable. You may be stuck and should get professional help.

If you grew up in a family that did not teach you to identify your feelings, you may need to learn now. You will also need to learn what to do about them. Don't be embarrassed. Simply begin now. Start with the feeling you wrote from the list.

▷ **Step 1:** Ask yourself the following:

When did I first feel this feeling? _____

_____

_____

How old was I? _____

What was I doing? _____

_____

_____

How did others around me react? _____

_____

_____

What did I need? _____

_____

▷ **Step 2:** As you look back at what was happening, how would you change the situation so you could have more power or control?

I would _____

_____

▷ **Step 3:** Recall a time when you felt powerful or successful. Let yourself experience this feeling fully. Now, apply the feeling to the above situation and see it coming out differently than it did the first time.

You can now use this approach with each feeling marked with a 1 or a 2 that you want to change. *Remember,* you don't need to change anything you don't want to.

Special information about specific feelings helps you to understand them better. Learning more about the feeling will help you be more effective in gaining control over it.

ANGER

What it is: A cover-up emotion. There is always another emotion under anger, one that makes you feel vulnerable in relation to having ADD.

What it does: It protects you.

What's underneath it: Fear, helplessness, frustration, or hopelessness.

What you can do to fix it: Find another way to protect yourself. Build your feelings of power. For example, learn to say "No." Or, stick to what you believe is right for you even if others tell you differently.

RAGE

What it is: Intense anger built up over a long period of time. If you were abused as a result of having ADD, you may experience rage.

What it does: It defends us from threats of harm.

What's underneath it: Terror, severe helplessness, abject hopelessness

What you can do to fix it: Work with a counselor who is trained in handling rage. Slowly, heal yourself in relation to the experiences that created the terror in the first place. Build your sense of powerfulness to defend yourself now.

NERVOUSNESS

What it is: A general state of anxious feelings. Insecurity about yourself and fear of doing something wrong. Many experiences of failure because of ADD can create nervousness.

What you can do to fix it: Tell yourself it is okay to make a mistake or be less than perfect. Practice. Gain experience.

SADNESS

What it is: A perfectly normal reaction to a loss. With ADD, it is the loss of potential.

What it does: It helps us express our grief.

What you can do to fix it: Let yourself express it. Cry, sigh, or otherwise discharge the feeling.

DEPRESSION

What it is: A deeply sad feeling of loss characterized by withdrawal, feelings of helplessness, hopelessness, lowered self-worth, changes in sleep and appetite, and a decrease in energy and activity level. If you have been keenly hurt because of having ADD or lost hope in achieving your dreams and potential, depression can result.

What it does: It signals the person that a loss has really happened.

What you can do to fix it: Talk with a friend, family member, or counselor. Move about even though you don't feel like it. Keep on a regular schedule with sleep and eating. Be self-nurturing. Consider medication.

RESENTMENT

What it is: Angry feelings that blame someone or something else in response to feeling hurt or injured. You may feel resentful toward the people who hurt you because of your ADD, even though they may have done so out of ignorance.

What it does: It attempts to push away feelings of hurt.

What is underneath it: Fear, helplessness, frustration, and hopelessness.

What you can do to fix it: Grieve the loss of your potential. Either talk or write to the person who hurt you and say how you were hurt. Then say that you believe it was done from ignorance without an intent to harm. Then forgive the person.

BOREDOM

What it is: A need for stimulation. It is characteristic of some people who have ADD.

What it does: It may mask depression. It may be a sign of trying to do jobs that do not use your intelligence or creativity.

What you can do to fix it: Assess the cause. Look for ways to add variety and interest to the task. Become creative. Set new goals.

FEAR

What it is: A reaction of helplessness to someone or something that can hurt you. Fear may be realistic or unrealistic. Being afraid that you cannot reach your potential with ADD is realistic if the ADD is untreated. The fear is unrealistic if it's treated.

What is does: It warns you of danger and that you need to be careful.

What you can do to fix it: Determine whether it is realistic. Ask, "Can I really be hurt by the danger?" If your fear is unrealistic (greater than the danger), discover when and how you learned to be afraid. Face the feared person or object as soon as possible. Take small steps in facing the fear. Ask for support from others in facing your fear. Be gentle with yourself.

ANXIETY

What it is: An outward manifestation of fear. A feeling of apprehension and tension about the outcome of an event or the feeling that something bad might happen. You may be anxious about the outcome of your ADD treatment, fearing that you will not be able to cope any better than before.

What it does: It distracts attention from a feared situation.

What's underneath it: Often anger that is unexpressed because of fear.

What you can do to fix it: Check to see whether you have unexpressed anger. Talk about your anger, resentment, and depression with a good listener. Take small steps to face the situation that is making you anxious. Surround yourself with support. Congratulate yourself on the small steps you take to overcome your anxiety. Medication may be indicated if you have considerable anxiety.

33

COMPULSIVITY

What it is: A rigid way of behaving. A strong impulse to carry out a behavior in a prescribed way, often repetitively. Some people with ADD have marked tendencies to be compulsive. It's either all or nothing.

What it does: It provides a sense of control. It also helps provide a structure that allows you to complete tasks.

What you can do to fix it: Milder forms of compulsivity may actually be useful to people who have ADD because they provide helpful structure. Having a strong impulse to be compulsive may indicate the need for medication. It is important to allow others to be more flexible if they wish or you may be perceived as controlling and your relationships may be hurt.

SHAME

What it is: The painful sense that there is something wrong with you; a strong feeling of worthlessness. A common feeling that develops when ADD is not diagnosed and treated early in life.

What it does: It creates low self-esteem, withdrawal from others, and fear of self-expression.

What you can do about it: Realize that there is a physiological reason for your difficulties. Know that it was outside of your control. Express your feelings about having ADD. Befriend the child part of you that suffered from having ADD. (See exercise page 19) Forgive yourself for thinking poorly about yourself. Forgive others who acted out of ignorance. Begin to assert your uniqueness.

GUILT

What it is: A feeling that you have done something wrong or that you have not done something that you should have done. Your behavior and your intentions don't match up and you are aware of it. Persons with ADD almost always experience guilt because of the scoldings and criticism of others and from comparisons to others. It's an attempt to roll back the clock to fix something that causes you pain, "If only I had studied harder, I would have passed." Feeling guilty that you didn't study harder creates the illusion that studying harder would have prevented your failure. In reality, if you could have studied harder, you would have.

What it does: It gives you a false sense of control that you can do something to make your situation better.

What's underneath it: Feelings of helplessness arising from a situation you can't control.

What you can do to fix it: Let yourself go through the grief process thoroughly. Accept the reality of what was. Begin now, changing your life as someone who is getting ADD under control.

EXCITEMENT

What it is: An increase in emotional activity that tends to create a greater flow of adrenalin. Excitement as the result of something special happening is normal. Excitement about something special that's going to happen is also normal. Excitement feels good, especially to people who have ADD. Needing excitement in order to feel good, however, can be an addiction that commonly accompanies ADD. Thrill seeking is an example.

What it does: It creates pleasurable feelings.

What you can do about it: Recognize the *urge.* Say, "My excitement addiction is acting up." Have something you can do instead of seeking the excitement. It could be breathing or meditation, calling a friend, going out for a run, or working out. After the urge subsides, ask yourself what happened before you felt the need. Determine the triggers that led up to the urge. Change your environment so you don't get into the situations that create stress or the urge in your life. Know that you can learn to curb your addiction to excitement.

▶ Bad Habits You've Developed

Feelings are expressed through behavior of some kind. Angry feelings may be communicated verbally, through a temper outburst, through fighting, or by self punishment. It is not unusual for people with ADD to have developed some bad habits in relation to the way feelings are expressed. Any such habits that you have learned can be changed. Let's take a look at your behavior so that you can decide if you need or want to change any of it.

Answer the following questions:

Do I have a temper that gets out of control sometimes?

_____ yes _____ no

Do I get into fights?

_____ yes _____ no

Am I accused of mouthing off when I don't agree with something?

_____ yes _____ no

Do I blame others when something goes wrong for me?

_____ yes _____ no

Do I abuse myself physically? (This includes eating improperly, drinking in excess, or wounding yourself.)

_____ yes _____ no

Do I put people down verbally?

_____ yes _____ no

Am I hypercritical of myself?

_____ yes _____ no

Do I scold myself when I make a mistake?

_____ yes _____ no

Do I sabotage myself by taking on too much?

_____ yes _____ no

Do I act impulsively, setting myself up for trouble?

_____ yes _____ no

Do I act impatiently, setting myself up to fail?

_____ yes _____ no

Work on the areas that you marked "yes." Be honest and patient with yourself. You are worth the time to change the habits that get in the way of your living a happy, healthy, life.

TEMPER

Though the tendency to have a bad temper is characteristic of many people who have ADD, it does not have to go undisciplined.

Ask yourself the following questions:

As a child, was I given what I wanted when I threw a fit?

_____ yes _____ no

As an adult, do I still get what I want by throwing a fit?

_____ yes _____ no

Does someone close to me give in to me when I lose my temper?

_____ yes _____ no

Do I find myself apologizing for my temper?

_____ yes _____ no

One of the biggest problems with using your temper to get what you want is that you pay a high price later. You are likely either to feel guilty or be punished, scolded, or criticized for your methods.

It's up to you to decide if you want to change. If you do, proceed.

▷ **Step 1:** Think of the last time you lost your temper.
▷ **Step 2:** Ask yourself what you were doing before you blew up. There will be typical problems that set you up for a temper outburst.
▷ **Step 3:** Go to the person involved and apologize for losing your temper. It doesn't matter if it was some time ago. You have to start somewhere and there is no time like the present.
▷ **Step 4:** Congratulate yourself on beginning to stop the process of losing your temper.
▷ **Step 5:** Ask that person to help you the next time you seem to be getting out of control. Agree on a signal such as the time-out signal used by referees in sporting events. When either of you makes the sign, agree to immediately back off so you can simmer down, thus short-circuiting your temper.

▷ **Step 6:** The next time you lose your temper, do the same thing listed in the first four steps. You will find that it takes you less time to remedy the situation each time. Soon you will begin to catch yourself while you are starting to fume. Finally you will catch yourself before you even blow up. It's only a matter of training.

▷ **Step 7:** Keep a sharp lookout for situations that tend to make you angry.

▷ **Step 8:** Find other ways to handle the situations so you do not need to feel so frustrated. For example, if your wife puts off balancing the checkbook or doesn't do it accurately, hire someone to do it or make a trade with someone who needs a skill you have.

▷ **Step 9:** Congratulate yourself on a job well done.

FIGHTING

Physical fighting or overreacting to someone touching or threatening you can become a habit. Choosing to pick a fight before you have exhausted all other ways of settling a situation is not constructive. You can still preserve your honor and find alternatives to getting in fights.

Ask yourself the following questions:

Have I gotten into any fights as a grown-up?

_____ yes _____ no

Did I try other ways to settle the problem?

_____ yes _____ no

Had I been drinking?

_____ yes _____ no

Can I think of strategies to solve problems other than fighting?

_____ yes _____ no

If you are now ready to change the habit of fighting first proceed.

▷ **Step 1:** If you answered "yes" to the question about drinking, you need to begin there.

38

▷ **Step 2:** It is important that you seek counseling in relation to your drinking habits. Get involved with Alcoholics Anonymous and/or a treatment program. You deserve to have a clean bill of health in this area.

▷ **Step 3:** Think through what preceded the fight. What were you doing? Did a lot of things happen that eventually added up to your getting in the fight or did it happen quickly.

▷ **Step 4:** It's imperative that you make a commitment to *talk* about whatever led up to the fight so you can train yourself to use your words instead of your fists. Find a buddy you can talk with any time.

▷ **Step 5:** If you got into the fight because someone grabbed you, like grabbing your arm to make a point, practice pulling away and backing off. Then sternly say, "Don't grab me. What do you want?" People with ADD are often especially sensitive to physical touching. You will know if this is you. There is no reason to make matters worse by getting out of control. Practice your reactions so you won't be caught off guard.

MOUTHING OFF

Spitting out a line of four-letter words or loudly blaming everyone and his ancestors for whatever you dislike is a habit that can be broken. Allowing yourself to get verbally out of control only makes others discount what you say. And since your words can be powerful allies in getting what you want, it is helpful to make the most of them.

Ask yourself:

Do I have a habit of swearing, *a lot?*

_____ yes   _____ no

Do I tend to swear when I am under stress?

_____ yes   _____ no

Do I verbally put down other people when I am startled or surprised?

_____ yes   _____ no

Do I call people names?

_____ yes   _____ no

These kinds of reactions to stress reduce your power to get your needs met. If you would like to raise your level of effectiveness, continue.

Be sure to separate the person from his behavior. That goes for you, too. You are not bad because you swear. The swearing *behavior* is what is bad or nonacceptable.

▷ **Step 1:** Think about the last time you mouthed off.
▷ **Step 2:** Ask yourself what you were feeling right before the words came out.
▷ **Step 3:** Write the words down below.
▷ **Step 4:** On the next line, write what you were feeling when you said them.
▷ **Step 5:** Next to the four-letter words, write words that you could substitute for them.
▷ **Step 6:** Now visualize the situation again and substitute the new words for the old four-letter ones as you respond to the situation.

Example:

You blankety-blank-blank	You scared me a lot.
	Don't do that again.
	(Yell if you need to.)
(The nonconstructive words)	(The new words)

It scared me a lot when the driver in front suddenly changed lanes. His driving is awful. He's not.
(What I was feeling)

Work the exercise through for yourself.

_____   _____
(The nonconstructive words)   (The new words)

_____

(What I was feeling)

Though changing your words will take some time, you can do it. At first, you will simply become aware of your mouthing off, but given time, you will begin to catch yourself. All that you have to do is be willing to listen to yourself and correct what comes out of your mouth.

SELF-PUNISHMENT

Rather than blaming others for what is causing you to feel stress, you may be blaming yourself. Scolding yourself and being hypercritical of yourself are two forms self-punishment can take. Calling yourself names is another. You don't deserve to be put down any more than another person does.

Remember: Your behavior is different from your self. Disliking something you've done is very different from disliking yourself.

Ask yourself:

Do I call myself names?

_____ yes _____ no

Do I criticize myself in my mind, saying things like this: "I should have studied harder. Then I could have gotten an 'A' instead of a 'B'." Do you use a scolding tone?

_____ yes _____ no

Do I feel like a little kid who is being scolded for having made a mistake?

_____ yes _____ no

Do I blame myself over and over again, saying things like this: "You're always doing dumb things. Won't you ever learn?"

_____ yes _____ no

Either never allowing yourself to feel good about your actions or criticizing every mistake you make does not help you do better next time.

Self-criticism is generally learned behavior. You learned it from

> ▷ another person in your family who was self-critical, in which case you copied the behavior.
> ▷ someone who criticized you *a lot* when you were growing up. Growing up, after all, is when you practiced the skills and abilities that you have now. If you hadn't made mistakes, you wouldn't have learned. Unfortunately, people with ADD were often scolded and criticized more than the average child.

It is time to reprogram yourself. If you are willing, proceed. (Extreme perfectionism may be biochemical and benefit from medication. See a physician for help.)

If you are perfectionist or self critical, try the following exercise.

▷ **Step 1:** Ask yourself, "Who else in my family was perfectionistic and self-critical?"

▷ **Step 2:** Write the name of the person here.

_____

▷ **Step 3:** Mentally, visualize yourself talking with that person. Say, "I realize you want to do things perfectly, but I want to experiment. That may mean that I will make mistakes. I will, however learn from my errors and not make you responsible for them. I hope you understand my being different from you."

▷ **Step 4:** Then forgive the person for trying to help in the wrong way.

▷ **Step 5:** Give yourself permission to make mistakes.

If the thought of making a mistake is very fearful, do the following exercise.

▷ **Step 1:** Let yourself make one mistake a day.

▷ **Step 2:** Make a note of the mistake.

▷ **Step 3:** Congratulate yourself for allowing yourself to have a learning experience.

▷ **Step 4:** Problem-solve to correct your mistake.

▷ **Step 5:** Fix the result of the mistake.

▷ **Step 6:** Congratulate yourself on the correction.

If you scold yourself for things you do, take the following steps:

▷ **Step 1:** Ask yourself who scolded you as a child.

▷ **Step 2:** Write the names of the people below. This may include family members, teachers, and coaches.

_____

_____

_____

_____

▷ **Step 3:** Write what they said below.

_____

_____

_____

_____

_____

▷ **Step 4:** Let the adult part of you tell the little child part of you that they were wrong to scold you. Write here what you want to say and how you feel.

_____

_____

_____

_____

▷ **Step 5:** Commit to protect the child part of you from now on. Write here what you want to say.

_____

▷ **Step 6:** Forgive the people who scolded you. They didn't know any better.

▷ **Step 7:** Forgive yourself.

SELF-SABOTAGE

Two common ways that people with ADD sabotage themselves is by:

▷ Agreeing to do things they don't want to do.

▷ Taking on too much at a time.

Ask yourself the following questions:

Do I try to be a nice guy by doing what others want?

_____ yes _____ no

Do I agree to things that I don't really feel like doing but feel I should do?

_____ yes _____ no

Am I afraid others won't like me if I don't do what they want?

_____ yes _____ no

Do I have big problems with time management?

_____ yes _____ no

Have I often agreed to do too many things at the same time?

_____ yes _____ no

43

Is it very hard for me to turn people down when they ask me to do things?

_____ yes _____ no

Taking on more than you can comfortably accomplish is a sure way to set yourself up to fail. If you find it difficult to organize tasks, set priorities, and manage time, you may end up angry at others or have them angry at you.

If you are ready to tackle these difficulties, proceed.

▷ **Step 1:** Make a commitment to yourself to do only what you want to do. Write your commitment below.

_____

_____

_____

_____

▷ **Step 2:** If you agree to something you don't want to do, own up to your error.

▷ **Step 3:** Tell the person that you made a mistake.

▷ **Step 4:** Offer to help the person problem-solve about what else can be done to meet their need.

▷ **Step 5:** Congratulate yourself on being honest.

If you misjudge the number of tasks you can accomplish in a certain amount of time so that you are in a frenzy trying to get them all done, consider the following:

▷ **Step 1:** Be honest with yourself about having taken on too much.

▷ **Step 2:** Ask for help. Either turn an entire task over to someone else, ask for help with part of the task, or ask for an extension of the deadline for the task.

▷ **Step 3:** Since the taking on of too many tasks is often a chronic problem, you may need to revise the way in which you agree to do things.

▷ **Step 4:** When you are asked to do something, *do not agree immediately!* Say, "Let me think about it. I'll let you know tomorrow." If the person tries to hurry you into a decision, say, "It wouldn't be fair for me to agree to something I might not be able to finish in a timely manner. If you need to know immediately, I'll have to say 'no.'"

▷ **Step 5:** Congratulate yourself on a job well done. You really are trainable!

Remember: Do not agree immediately.

If you have time management problems, the following will help.

▷ **Step 1:** Ask someone to sit down with you and plan out a weekly schedule. Be sure to allow enough time for driving to appointments, eating lunch, and watching TV. Together you can come up with a way to keep a schedule that will help you. (In the appendix there are some different kinds of scheduling sheets for you to try.)

▷ **Step 2:** Next, try to make out your own schedule using the same forms and methods you tried earlier.

▷ **Step 3:** Set a definite time every week to lay out next week's schedule.

▷ **Step 4:** Commit to always looking at your schedule before agreeing to any jobs or appointments.

▷ **Step 5:** If someone kids you about keeping a schedule, say, "That's okay. I stay out of lot more trouble since I got myself organized."

IMPULSIVITY

When you act without thinking, you act impulsively. There is no planning or taking responsibility for the outgrowth of your act.

Underneath all impulsive behavior is fear:

▷ Fear that our needs will not get met.

▷ Fear that we will not be able to feel okay unless we have whatever we think and believe will make us feel satisfied.

Ask yourself the following:

Do I frequently act without thinking?

_____ yes   _____ no

Do I get into trouble for impulsive behavior?

_____ yes   _____ no

Am I told, "You never seem to think things through"?

_____ yes   _____ no

Do I feel confident that I can get what I want even if it takes time?

_____ yes   _____ no

Do I have an addiction?

_____ yes _____ no

Do I take responsibility for the results of my behavior?

_____ yes _____ no

Being afraid that you won't be able to get your important needs met is very frightening. Unless you trust that they will get met or you have the power to get them met, you are likely to act impulsively.

Impulses mask hidden needs. Those needs may be in direct opposition to your goals. For example, your goal may be to save money but your need is to feel fulfilled. Buying something you want makes you feel fulfilled. But when you buy something, you have undermined your goal to save.

Ask yourself the following:

What makes me feel good? Write it below.

_____

_____

_____

_____

What price do I pay for using this to feel good?

_____

_____

_____

_____

_____

What are some other ways I can feel good?

_____

_____

_____

_____

_____

If you have a full-fledged addiction, you will probably need the help of a twelve-step program. You will be surprised that you can get beyond your addiction *and* feel good inside.

It is possible to curb your impulses, replacing them with more suitable ways to get your needs met at a much lower cost. If you are willing to change, proceed.

▷ **Step 1:** List your impulses below.

_____

_____

_____

▷ **Step 2:** Choose one to work with here. Write it down.

_____

▷ **Step 3:** What did you want to feel by fulfilling the impulse?

_____

_____

▷ **Step 4:** What are you afraid of if you don't act impulsively?

_____

_____

▷ **Step 5:** What makes you afraid that you cannot feel good except through the use of your impulsive behavior?

_____

_____

▷ **Step 6:** Make a list of other ways to get your need met. **Remember:** Whatever you feel or need is legitimate. How you express or try to fulfill the need is what gets changed, not the need.

_____

_____

_____

▷ **Step 7:** Realize that you can and will get what you need. It is only necessary to plan how to get your need met so that you don't have to pay dearly for the results you get. And you can actually get better results with responsible planning.

▷ **Step 8:** If you get stuck, or are unable to figure out anything to help you meet your need, begin to reach out to others. Several people working together will bring new viewpoints and solutions to your problem.

▷ **Step 9:** The key to breaking the habit of impulsivity is practice. Train yourself to stop, listen, and think before you act.

IMPATIENCE

The fear that you will not acquire what you want underlies impatience. When you have difficulty trusting that your needs will get met, you are likely to experience impatience.

Ask yourself the following:

Were my needs met in a timely manner when I was young?

_____ yes _____ no

Did it seem forever until I felt relief?

_____ yes _____ no

Did someone misuse their power or control in relation to me?

_____ yes _____ no

Do I feel as if no one was on my side?

_____ yes _____ no

Did I feel helpless or alone in trying to get my needs met?

_____ yes _____ no

Do I have creative ways to pass time until I get what I want?

_____ yes _____ no

Having creative ways to pass time and having the inner security to know that you will get what you need will help you to exercise patience. It is the gift that trust brings. Expecting to become patient by simply telling yourself to be patient is not realistic. Rather, it is necessary to build the strengths from which patience develops.

If you are ready to build a foundation for patience, proceed.

▷ **Step 1:** Initially seek reassurance from outside of yourself. Talk with someone who is farther down the road than you: a mentor who supports and reassures you but not one who does your job for you.

▷ **Step 2:** You are the one who will figure out new ways to pass the time until what you want happens. List ten ways to spend your time waiting. (Later it won't even seem like waiting, but for now, it's okay to think of it that way.)

_____

_____

_____

_____

_____

_____

_____

_____

_____

_____

▷ **Step 3:** Hang your list of ten on the wall where you can see it, or carry it in your billfold. Whenever you become impatient, feel as if time is moving too slowly, or feel that you can't stand to wait any longer, pull the list out and pick one of the ten. You might even want to add a little sport to this. Close your eyes and point with one finger, picking one blind. Why not?

▷ **Step 4:** Commit to follow through with the distraction you picked.

▷ **Step 5:** When you feel stronger, you can make up new distractions at the time you are feeling the urgency.

▷ **Step 6:** Each time you succeed in following through on your commitment, congratulate yourself for a job well done.

▷ **Step 7:** Notice that you were actually able to wait. See, you _are_ developing patience. Trust yourself and your inner creative resources and strength. That's what patience is all about.

Know that you have the ability to develop many new, constructive habits. Believe in yourself and you will succeed in becoming the wonderful person you were always meant to be. Congratulations.

Chapter 4

Essential Skills

▶ Taking Control: Planning Ahead

Waiting until the last minute to do a project is characteristic of many people who have ADD. You can train yourself, however, to plan ahead so that you can complete things in a timely manner.

What you can do: Learn to plan ahead.

How you do it:

▷ **Step 1:** Get a month-long calendar.

▷ **Step 2:** Mark in any deadlines you know about now.

▷ **Step 3:** As soon as a deadline is announced, mark it in.

▷ **Step 4:** Figure out how long it will take you to complete the project.

▷ **Step 5:** Count back that number of days and mark *start*. Notice that you are not asked to add a couple of days. *There is nothing wrong with working under pressure.* It often helps people with ADD to focus their attention. The only constraint is that you not create chaos because you didn't allow enough time. You, and only you, are responsible for the completion of the project on time. You will learn to judge time by taking responsibility for the completion of projects yourself.

▷ **Step 6:** Begin the project.

▷ **Step 7:** Check once or twice a day to see how you are coming. The frequency depends upon how much reinforcement you want to give yourself. Congratulate yourself for the amount of work you have completed when you check. *Do not put attention on the work you do not accomplish.* Place a check here for each segment of the work you complete.

51

Segment 1 _____   Segment 2 _____   Segment 3 _____

Segment 4 _____   Segment 5 _____   Segment 6 _____

Segment 7 _____   Segment 8 _____

▷ **Step 8:** Congratulate yourself for completing the entire project in a timely manner. Place a check on this line when you complete it. _____

▶ Transitions

Transitions are typically difficult for people who have ADD. They often have difficulty changing from one activity to another. Though it may take you time to get started on an activity, once the activity is begun, you may find it difficult to stop the activity.

What you can do: Learn to change from activity to activity in a timely manner.

How you can do it:

▷ **Step 1:** Pick a time to start an activity.
▷ **Step 2:** Decide how long you want or need to spend on the activity.
▷ **Step 3:** Stick to that time whether you are ready or not.
▷ **Step 4:** Set a timer or set the alarm on your watch for the amount of time you are willing to spend on the project.
▷ **Step 5:** Stop the activity the moment the alarm goes off. No delays. No excuses. No extra minutes.
▷ **Step 6:** Mark down the time.
▷ **Step 7:** Reset your alarm or timer so you are alerted to when you may return to the project. (Do this for things you like to do as well as things you don't much like to do.)
▷ **Step 8:** Start the next stage when your timer goes off. No delays. No excuses. No extra minutes.
▷ **Step 9:** Congratulate yourself.
▷ **Step 10:** Revise your self-image. Label yourself as someone who *can* manage time.

▶ Working Out a Schedule

Every person with ADD has a preferred approach to scheduling. It is important that you use the method that works best for you. There is not a better or worse way, only different ways to schedule time. Here are some typical types of schedules.

- ▷ The blank page method.
- ▷ Plan for the day.
- ▷ Plan for the week.
- ▷ Having someone else make your plan.
- ▷ The Dictaphone method.
- ▷ The computer-program method.

Put a check by any methods you want to try. You may choose as many as you want. For the sake of variety, you may want to use more than one, changing from time to time. You can also use a combination.

THE BLANK PAGE METHOD

▷ **Step 1:** Set aside the same time each day to work out your schedule.

▷ **Step 2:** Get out a blank piece of paper.

▷ **Step 3:** Write down all the things you can think of that you need or want to do that day. Don't worry initially about organizing them.

▷ **Step 4:** Take a deep breath.

▷ **Step 5:** Set priorities. Which needs to be done first, second, third? Number them 1, 2, etc. Or you may wish to underline in one color the *have to's*. Do what feels good to you.

▷ **Step 6:** Decide if you want to order them neatly on a separate sheet of paper. You don't have to in order to be successful.

▷ **Step 7:** Make sure the list is in plain sight. Pin the paper on the wall or put it in front of you on your desk.

▷ **Step 8:** Cross out each item as it is completed.

▷ **Step 9:** Congratulate yourself for each completed item.

▷ **Step 10:** Feel free to change the items around as the day proceeds unless that will get you off track. Do what works best for you. Also feel free to stop for a break using the method outlined on the previous page.

PLAN FOR THE DAY

▷ **Step 1:** Get a ready-made appointment book or use sheets like the one on page 174. Feel free to be creative by designing your own.

▷ **Step 2:** Work with your schedule at the same time daily. Frequently, the first thing in the morning or the last thing at the end of your day is the best, but remember that you can change any instructions given here so that they fit your preferences.

▷ **Step 3:** Put in the obligations you have. Highlight the important items. Colored markers often work well for this.

▷ **Step 4:** Put in the times you want to do something for yourself. Use a different color to mark these.

▷ **Step 5:** Check or cross out items as you complete them.

▷ **Step 6:** Congratulate yourself.

PLAN FOR THE WEEK

▷ **Step 1:** At the same time weekly, lay out what you know are standing commitments. Use the schedule (page 174) as a sample.

▷ **Step 2:** Add time out for yourself. Some people with ADD do better if they stay on the same basic schedule every day. Others need variety so they won't get bored. Do what fits you best.

▷ **Step 3:** Fill in one project that you have been putting off. Either break it into chunks that are spread throughout the week or set aside one day for the project. Do what fits you best.

▷ **Step 4:** Look back over your schedule. Mark all *have to's* with a red underliner. Do this first each day.

▷ **Step 5:** Check off your accomplishments as the day goes by.

▷ **Step 6:** Revise your schedule as needed with additions or deletions.

▷ **Step 7:** Congratulate yourself on a job well done.

HAVING SOMEONE ELSE MAKE YOUR SCHEDULE

Making a trade with someone else to give you a helping hand with your schedule is perfectly all right. You can trade money for secretarial time. You can trade a skill. All it takes is two people agreeing to make a deal.

What do you have to trade? Check below the things you have to trade.

_____ 1. *Money*

How much would I be willing to spend? _____

_____ 2. *Skills*

What skills do I have to offer? _____

_____

_____ 3. *Time*

How much time do I have to give? _____

_____

4. Other _____

_____

Now you are ready to begin working with the other person.

▷ **Step 1:** Tell the other person what you need to get done.
▷ **Step 2:** Let the person make suggestions.
▷ **Step 3:** Approve the suggestions or let the person know of changes you would like made.

You may want a standard schedule outline that stays the same so that your helper can simply do your scheduling within that framework. All you have to do is show up on time. If you begin to have trouble with arriving on time, go to the next step.

▷ **Step 4:** Have a meeting with your helper and problem-solve the difficulty. You probably have failed to schedule in the amount of time needed for one or more activities, such as travel time or relaxation time, or you have let yourself get distracted by things you'd rather do. On the other hand, you may be avoiding something you don't want to do or are afraid to do.
▷ **Step 5:** Problem-solve the difficulty. Be honest. Be sure you mean to do what you have agreed to do. It's very difficult to get ourselves to do anything we really don't want to do.

If you are really afraid of a task or feel inadequate to accomplish it, you may need to visit a counselor, teacher, or mentor so you can get past the difficulty.

THE DICTAPHONE METHOD

Training yourself to use a Dictaphone may be the smartest move you have ever made. It usually requires a good secretarial person or staff to transcribe and implement the directions you give on your recorder.

▷ **Step 1:** Begin to use a Dictaphone to give directions to your secretary. Do this first thing in the morning or last thing in the day.
▷ **Step 2:** Have it at home and record ideas you have away from work.
▷ **Step 3:** When you are working, begin to give directions for your secretary to follow through on.
▷ **Step 4:** Give that person the tape at the same time daily.
▷ **Step 5:** Have the person place the completed items on your desk the next day. Go over them with your Dictaphone in hand so you can note any corrections or instructions for follow-through.
▷ **Step 6:** Congratulate yourself and the other person on a job well done.

THE COMPUTER PROGRAM METHOD

Keeping your schedule on your computer is a good idea if you are particularly drawn to using computers. Many people with ADD are, so this method may fit easily into your desire to work out computer programs, try out new software, or simply play games.

▷ **Step 1:** When you first sit down at the computer, pull up the scheduling program on the screen.

▷ **Step 2:** Check how much you accomplished that day and give yourself a pat on the back.

▷ **Step 3:** Pull up tomorrow's schedule. Make revisions and additions. If it is the first of the week, you may want to go ahead and lay the rest of the week out for yourself.

▷ **Step 4:** When you have finished polishing your schedule, reward yourself with a game or other computer activity that you enjoy, knowing you did a good job.

Although scheduling may not be your favorite activity, you can learn to make one and live by it. More power to you.

H.A.L.T.

Taken from twelve-step programs, H.A.L.T. identifies common triggers that can sabotage your attempts at taking control of your life.

"H" stands for hungry.

When you are hungry, your energy will be low and you are more likely to have poor judgment or do things without thinking. Be sure you plan regular times for meals and/or snacking into your schedule.

"A" stands for angry.

When you are angry, you are likely to do things for the wrong reasons, taking your anger out on others or yourself. Such displacement will get you off track, sabotaging your efforts to take control of your life. Plan in time to resolve angry feelings. Do not let them build up. If you are angry a lot of the time, work through the section on page 35. Don't hesitate to see a counselor to help with this one.

"L" stands for lonely.

Feeling lonely is a distraction that takes your attention away from the planned schedule you developed at an earlier time. Seeking companionship or a sense of belonging is an emotional need that we all have. Be sure to schedule time in for meeting those needs.

"T" stands for tired.

When tiredness hits, our judgment goes out the window quickly. Part of making a schedule that works includes allowing sufficient time to rest and recuperate. If you are a night owl, plan some rest time during the day.

Go back to your schedule. Add time for these common pitfalls.

KNOW YOUR LIMITS

To feel comfortable and secure in your daily life, it is critical that you establish boundaries. Frequently a person with ADD spends a lot of time trying to do what is expected or what someone else thinks should be done. Yet to be successful and happy, you must establish the limits within which you are willing to work and live. This includes knowing what you will and won't do as well as what you can and can't do.

Ask yourself the following questions:

Do I sometimes let other people run over me?

_____ yes   _____ no

Do I let someone else tell me what to do and how to do it?

_____ yes   _____ no

Am I always trying to please someone else?

_____ yes   _____ no

Do I trust my own judgment?

_____ yes   _____ no

Do I do what I want to do?

_____ yes   _____ no

Am I able to tell others "No"?

_____ yes   _____ no

Limits provide clear definition. They identify how you spend your time, what you do, and the manner in which you do it. If you are ready to take charge of your time and space, you are ready to learn more about setting your limits. In this case, proceed.

Get in touch with your feelings.

57

▷ **Step 1:** For the rest of the day, keep track of how you feel about everything you do.

▷ **Step 2:** Ask yourself, "Do I like what I am doing? Am I happy doing what I am doing? Am I doing it the way I want to do it?"

▷ **Step 3:** You may want to keep a log listing what you are doing. Place a plus mark by the things you like. Put a minus by those you dislike. Then, at the end of the day, add the signs up. If you have more minuses than pluses, you may wish to take better control of your life.

▷ **Step 4:** Make a list of things you want to change.

So far, so good. You now know how you feel about some of the things in your life. If you would like to actually change them, proceed.

Set your limits.

▷ **Step 1:** Start with something small. For example, your spouse may want you to help fold the laundry but wants you to fold the towels in thirds lengthwise and then in half across. You prefer to fold them in half and then half again. You feel very irritable every time she corrects the way you do it and generally you pick a fight when you do the laundry.

▷ **Step 2:** Become clear in your mind about what you will and won't do.

▷ **Step 3:** At another time, when there is no laundry to be done, ask your wife to meet with you because you have something you want to talk with her about. Do not piggyback this discussion onto anything else you are doing. Also, don't bring it up when either of you is in a hurry.

▷ **Step 4:** Prepare for the meeting by thinking through what you are and are not willing to do. Figure out if and how much you are willing to compromise.

▷ **Step 5:** Tell your wife that you respect her approach to folding the clothes but that you have a different approach. Be careful not to become scolding. Check to be sure that you feel that your way is not better or worse than hers, only different.

▷ **Step 6:** Then set the limit. You may choose to say that you are willing to fold the towels your way, but that if you do, you do not want to be corrected or scolded. Tell her that if that is not acceptable, you will simply leave the towels for her to fold.

▷ **Step 7:** Do not be pressured into going against what you feel is best. If she pressures you, tell her calmly that you do not want to fight and that your relationship is worth protecting, so you won't do something that doesn't feel good to you.

▷ **Step 8:** Congratulate yourself. You've taken major steps toward keeping your relationship with your wife healthy. You also have demonstrated self control. (Later, we'll talk about consensus.)

Know when to say "No." When it comes to limits, this is the most important word you will ever learn. The ability to say "No" in ways that are not offensive is a skill you deserve to have. It only takes practice.

▷ **Step 1:** Think of a situation recently that you encountered when you agreed to do something that you didn't want to do. For example, the mothers' club at school may have asked you to bake cookies for the meeting. You already had too much to do but you said "Yes" for fear the caller would think poorly of you. Afterwards you felt angry about baking the cookies and resentful that the person had asked you.

▷ **Step 2:** Acknowledge to yourself that you got into the situation because you failed to follow your feelings. You failed to say "No." It wasn't the other person's fault. You must take responsibility for the mess you allowed yourself to get in.

▷ **Step 3:** Make a commitment to yourself that you will say "No" the next time you are asked to do something that you don't want to do or that would put you under stress.

▷ **Step 4:** Visualize a person who might ask for something you don't want to give. See yourself saying, "No, I won't be able to do that." Realize you don't need to give reasons for why you won't do it. Variations of "No" include "I'm sorry I won't be able to do it," "I can't let myself commit to anything else now," or "I wish I could help you, but I'm not able to."

▷ **Step 5:** Be sure to say "No" when you are under much stress or there is a lot of change in your life. Be sure that the loudest request does not get your attention so that you end up ignoring requests from people who are less demanding. Be sure you don't shortchange family members with whom you feel safe and secure. Are you tempted to put off the requests of those you are close to because it seems safe to do so while agreeing to requests from acquaintances who mean less to you?

► The "Uh-huh" Syndrome

Many people with ADD have a bad habit of vocalizing "Uh-huh" when asked to do something only to fail to follow through with what seemed to be a commitment. Many a friend or spouse has become angry when disappointed by the lack of completion of a project or agreement, saying, "But you *said* you'd do it!"

Ask yourself the following questions:

Have you been accused of not listening?

_____ yes   _____ no

Do other people get angry at you, saying you don't follow through on a promise?

_____ yes   _____ no

Do you tend to agree to things so others won't get angry at you?

_____ yes   _____ no

Are you afraid of letting people down?

_____ yes   _____ no

The more "Yes" answers you gave, the more likely it is that you are to be susceptible to the "Uh-huh" syndrome. It creates major problems in relationships because people count on you to do what you seemingly have committed to do. There are two stages to remedying the situation.

Stage One: You must become aware that you are saying "Uh-huh" when you say it.

▷ **Step 1:** Ask a friend or spouse to work with you.
▷ **Step 2:** Tell the person that you are trying to break a habit and that you want to become aware of when you say "Uh-huh." Ask the person to give you a sign when you say it so that you become aware.
▷ **Step 3:** Each time you become aware of saying "Uh-huh," stop and repeat what was asked of you.
▷ **Step 4:** Ask yourself whether you really *want* to do what you said "Uh-huh" to.

It is imperative that you only agree to what you want. Do not agree to anything because you are afraid someone will get angry with you.

Sometimes people with ADD say "Uh-huh" when they want to simply acknowledge that they hear the other person talking. It does not necessarily mean that they are agreeing or committing to do something.

Stage Two: Translating the vocal agreement into action takes a second, conscious commitment to do more than listen. Besides listening, you must actually take responsibility to implement whatever you agreed to do.

▷ **Step 1:** After you have stopped yourself in order to determine whether you really want to do what you said "Uh-huh" to, you need to think.

▷ **Step 2:** Make a conscious decision that you are willing to take action.

▷ **Step 3:** Make a plan of action. Include a timetable for completion of the task.

▷ **Step 4:** Follow through with what you have agreed to do.

▷ **Step 5:** Feel good about having learned a new skill.

Anyone involved with a person who has ADD must check in with that person when hearing "Uh-huh" to be sure that the intent is in place to complete the task. There is no point in setting both of you up for disappointment and resentment.

▶ Asking for Help

One of the most important skills anyone with ADD can learn is how to ask for help. Often the skill has not been developed, partly because early school years may have been marked by attempts to avoid attention. Or perhaps, when you did ask, you were scolded for not having paid attention the first time. It wouldn't have taken you long to learn to stay silent.

Ask yourself the following questions:

When I was a child, was I scolded for asking for clarification on assignments?

_____ yes   _____ no

Did all the other kids seem to catch on faster than I did?

_____ yes   _____ no

Do I try to do everything myself now so that I don't have to ask for help?

_____ yes   _____ no

61

Am I embarrassed if I have to ask for help?

_____ yes _____ no

On the job, do I try to hide inadequacies?

_____ yes _____ no

Do I feel bad about myself because I don't learn quickly enough?

_____ yes ___ no

Now it is time to work on changing a habit that will restrict your effectiveness. The more "yes" responses you have, the more difficult it may be to commit to change. But all you have to do is give yourself permission. Then gather your courage to make the change. Ready? Check here if you're ready to proceed.

_____ yes

GIVE YOURSELF PERMISSION

▷ **Step 1:** Think back about when and where you learned that it was unsafe or embarrassing or uncomfortable to ask for help.

▷ **Step 2:** As you remember a particular scene, freeze-frame the moment in your mind.

▷ **Step 3:** Now, ask yourself what you needed in the way of help.

▷ **Step 4:** Say to yourself, "It's okay to ask for help. The child needed help, and I'm going to give it to him."

▷ **Step 5:** Then say the words that would have provided help to the child.

▷ **Step 6:** Tell the child that it is okay to ask for help anytime he or she needs or wants it.

▷ **Step 7:** Now, say to your adult self, "It's okay to ask for help anytime I need it."

COMMUNICATE CLEARLY

It is important to communicate clearly and concisely when you are asking for help. Rambling sentences and too many verbal side journeys will tend to reduce the effectiveness of the help you obtain because

    1. this may diminish the person's interest.

2. it may make it difficult for the person to know what you want.
3. it wastes everyone's valuable time.

You will find the following steps helpful in raising the effectiveness of your communication.

▷ **Step 1:** Practice making "I" statements.

"I would appreciate a few minutes of your time."

"I need a helping hand with my backyard fence. Would you be able to help me next Saturday?"

Even if you forgot until the last minute that you needed to get printed material ready for a workshop, say, "I forgot to get the material ready for Monday's workshop. I'll understand if you have other plans, but I want to ask if you could help me. It will take about an hour."

▷ **Step 2:** Do *not* assume the person will be able to help you just because you ask. (This is especially true of personal relationships.) *Asking isn't assuming.*

▷ **Step 3:** Before speaking to the person, be clear about exactly what you want to get. Practice being concise. Change the following to be more concise.

"My mother-in-law is coming and it's very important that I finish painting the bedroom that she is going to use. You know, the one that has the pink wallpaper at the head of the bed. I was going to do it on Friday but I have to take my kids to a birthday party over at their cousins so I guess the only time left is Saturday. I sure hope you can help me; otherwise I don't know what I will do."

_____

_____

_____

All you really need to say is: "I need help painting a bedroom. Are you available for two hours on Saturday?"

GATHER YOUR COURAGE

▷ **Step 1:** Think about something in your current life that you need help with. It might be a project, or some information that you need such as how you can obtain help at school with your studies because of your ADD. It could be emotional support or skills to use in communicating to your spouse.

I plan to ask for the following help:

_____

_____

_____

▷ **Step 2:** Next, take a deep breath.

▷ **Step 3:** Remind yourself that it is *smart* to ask for help.

▷ **Step 4:** Now, choose the person you want to seek help from.

I will ask help from (write the person's name or title) _____

_____

▷ **Step 5:** Decide whether you will call the person or make a personal contact.

I will _____

▷ **Step 6:** List the question or questions you want to ask. (Be specific)

I will ask the person to _____

_____

_____

_____

▷ **Step 7:** Estimate how much time you will need from the person.

I estimate it will take _____ time.

▷ **Step 8:** Ask for that amount of time. "Honey, could you help me a minute?" If you need an appointment, say, "I would like an appointment for one hour with you, please."

▷ **Step 9:** When you get it, mark the time down in your schedule immediately.

My appointment time is _____

▷ **Step 10:** The results of my meeting or contact are

_____

_____

_____

_____

▷ **Step 11:** Congratulate yourself on a job well done. You have demonstrated the courage to ask for help.

SAYING "THANK YOU"

There are many ways to say "Thank you." The most common and effective way is to simply say the words. It is not necessary to embellish your thank you with a lot of flowery words. *Keep it simple* and don't repeat yourself even though your gratitude may be great.

In the hustle-bustle of the modern world, the time it takes to write thank you notes makes them special.

Giving an *unsolicited special gift* to someone is great. A home-cooked pan of brownies for a busy executive may prove more valuable than you would ever guess.

Make a trade. Trading trips to drop the car off for service or picking up and delivering each other to the airport are exchanges that work well in today's world. These are the kinds of things that people do for each other.

► Networking

Networking is a process of connecting with other people who can help you achieve your goals. In turn you probably will be able to help them achieve theirs. But often the process is not a direct one in which you know going into a meeting what you will gain. Rather, it is more like scattering seed on the wind. You can count on some of them growing but you can't tell which ones they will be.

Principles of Networking

> ▷ Meet as many people as you can.
> ▷ Share with them what you are doing and what you are interested in.
> ▷ Find out what they are doing and what they are interested in.
> ▷ Look for opportunities to help them meet their goals.
> ▷ Give them something, such as a business card, to remember you by.
> ▷ Reestablish contact with them periodically.
> ▷ Keep them up to date on what you are doing.
> ▷ Be sure to say "Thank you."

The steps to networking are easy, yet if you have never been exposed to them, you may not know what to do or how to do it. If you would like to learn, proceed.

▶ How to Network

MEET AS MANY PEOPLE AS YOU CAN

▷ **Step 1:** Principle: You will find people to network with everywhere.

Strategy: Network with everyone you come in contact with. Even though you may be building a new dry-cleaning business, you may find just the resource you need at your child's soccer game.

▷ **Step 2:** Principle: Talk conversationally, not as a sales person.

Strategy: Avoid trying to *do business.* Rather, tell anecdotes, report interesting occurrences, and ask simple questions.

Examples:

Anecdote—"The other day, right after I received the first video, hot off the press, I realized I'd forgotten to have the address printed on the jacket. So much for inexperience!"

Interesting occurrences—"I discovered the most interesting thing last week. During the recording of my new video the microphones picked up some unwanted sound. But the producer was able to take it out. Isn't technology wonderful?"

Simple question—"Do you know anyone who does video packaging?"

Each of these examples conveys the information that I have a new video or steers the conversation around to a discussion in which information could be shared, yet none of them is a sales pitch that might be offensive or inappropriate. You will be able to discover other people who have an interest in videos or know someone who knows someone who might be a good contact.

▷ **Step 3:** Get each person's business card, address, or phone number and file it when you get home.

▷ **Step 4:** Trust your judgment about people you meet. If you like someone but have no idea how you can help one another, pursue the relationship anyway. Sooner or later you will discover a way to assist one another.

Share with others what you are doing.
Share with others what you are interested in.

Part of networking involves making yourself known to others. That includes what you are doing and what you are interested in. By sharing these aspects of yourself, you will imprint who you are and what you stand for on the other person's mind. Then, in the future when the person has a need that relates to something you can do, you will receive a call. The call may translate into a sale, a trade, or something else of interest to you.

Write things you are doing: jobs, projects, roles, etc.

_____   _____

_____   _____

_____   _____

_____   _____

Write interests that you have.

_____   _____

_____   _____

_____   _____

_____   _____

Now you have a beginning list of conversation items you can share.

Find out what others are doing.
Find out what others are interested in.

▷ **Step 1:** Think of someone you know casually.
▷ **Step 2:** List below what you already know about the person.

What the person is doing.

_____

_____

_____

_____

What the person is interested in.

_____

_____

_____

_____

▷ **Step 3:** The next time you spend time with the person, make a point of learning more about what that person is doing and what the person is interested in.

▷ **Step 4:** If you want, write down what you have discovered. Or you may just want to keep the information in your mind. You'll know what fits you best.

Look for opportunities to help the person achieve a goal.

▷ **Step 1:** Pick one or several people to observe during the next week. Watch for opportunities to help them achieve a goal.

▷ **Step 2:** When you observe one, ask the person whether he or she would like the help. You might say, "I ran across an outlet for galvanized pipe. Would you be interested in the name?" Even though you think your information is valuable, do not assume it is wanted. It may be, but be respectful.

▷ **Step 3:** You might want to inquire whether further scouting on your part is useful. "Would you like me to keep my eyes open for other sources of pipe?" Listen for the answer. The person may tell you that there is no longer a need for such a resource. This way you will not waste your time.

GIVE A REMINDER

Examples of ways to leave a reminder about yourself include the following:

▷ A business card
▷ An exchange of phone numbers on pieces of note paper.
▷ A telephone call at a later date.
▷ A note mailed shortly after your meeting saying how nice it was to talk.
▷ An invitation to something.
▷ A greeting card or holiday card.

Check the ways that sound good to you.

Reestablish contact periodically.
Keep others up to date.
Say "thanks."

From time to time over the years, it is useful to reestablish contact with people you knew previously. Playing catch-up is interesting and often people discover they have new interests in common. This can be done

▷ in person
▷ over the phone
▷ in writing

Think of three people you haven't connected with for over a year. Use one of the three ways listed above to reconnect. Write the person's name below and the way you choose to reconnect.

1. _____   _____
2. _____   _____
3. _____   _____

If the contact is made in person or over the phone, say, "Is this a good time to talk? I'd like to play catch-up." Communicate in a friendly manner, sharing the changes that have occurred in your life. Mention old interests that you still have and generally update the person about you and your life. Then ask about that person's life.

If any specific assistance comes out of the contact, be sure to say, "Thank you. I appreciate it."

If you receive a catch-up letter from someone and it is just not a good time for you to respond, drop a quick note saying so and that you will write more when you can.

Networking is a valuable tool of the twenty-first century. Most jobs are found through networking. Many business deals are made through networking and, often, friendships and interests of value are discovered through networking. Enjoy the use of it.

▶ Getting Rid of the "Shoulds"

Part of learning to handle ADD includes being certain that you are living with values of your own choosing rather than values you were taught that you **should** have.

Are Your Values Your Own?

Value is defined as

> ▷ worth
> ▷ merit
> ▷ importance

Values include those behaviors and beliefs about ourselves and life that we hold in high regard.

Values are important when you

> ▷ make decisions
> ▷ want to change what you are doing
> ▷ make a commitment to take action

In order to do anything, we must believe it is the **right** thing for us to do. We then give ourselves permission to do it.

However, some of our beliefs are not really our own. They are carried over from our childhood, and we experience them as "shoulds." (For example: "I should be polite at all times," "I should work first and play second," or "I should do unpleasant tasks conscientiously, no matter how hard they are.")

Anytime you try to do something you think you **should** do but don't really want to do, you will feel **resentful.**

List the things you do that make you feel resentful.

_____

_____

_____

_____

Anytime you do *not* do something you think you **should** do, you will feel **guilty.**

Make a list of the things you feel guilty about.

_____

_____

_____

_____

Do Only What You Believe Is Right for You

Agreeing to do something because you feel you **should**

  ▷ leads to failure.
  ▷ makes you sabotage the things you are trying to do.
  ▷ often makes you appear irresponsible because, since you feel resentful, you often procrastinate or do a sloppy job.
  ▷ makes you feel angry at the person you think expects your "should" behavior.

Since living with shoulds is nonconstructive, learn how to change "shoulds" to "wants."When you do things you want to do, you will not feel resentful and guilty and are likely to do a good job and feel good about yourself.

Go to the previous page and select the "shoulds" that you would like to change to "wants." Write them here.

_____

_____

_____

_____

There are two kinds of "shoulds":

1. Surface "shoulds"
2. Deeply rooted "shoulds"

Surface "shoulds" come from values that you haven't thought about one way or the other. They are behind the behaviors that you do automatically and habitually. However, when you become aware of your behavior, you are easily able to change in favor of a new way of doing things.

For example: You may have always celebrated New Year's with a favorite food but when your spouse says she's tired of it, you realize it does not bother you to change. You simply never thought of it before.

Deeply rooted "shoulds," on the other hand, are more difficult to change because they form a part of your identity, are surrounded by a great deal of emotion, and were reinforced throughout your childhood.

THE SHORT METHOD OF CHANGING "SHOULDS" TO "WANTS"

To change a surface value from a "should" to a "want," first, try the short method. Select one "should" from the previous page.

For example: You have cut the grass since you were fourteen years old. You hate cutting the grass and feel resentful that you have to do it now that you are married. You took it for granted when you got married that you would be the one to cut it. You never really stopped to think that you might do it differently.

▷ **Step 1:** Ask yourself whether you want to cut the grass.

_____ yes _____ no

▷ **Step 2:** If your answer is "no," ask yourself if you would be willing to look for an alternative.

_____ yes _____ no

▷ **Step 3:** If your answer is "yes," list alternatives. For example:
   ▷ Your wife might be willing to cut the grass, so she could do it.
   ▷ Your child might love to have a way to earn some money. You could start teaching him.
   ▷ You could hire someone to do it.

▷ **Step 4:** Consider the alternatives.

Then decide.

| I *choose* to cut the grass myself as I always have. | I *choose* a new way to get the grass cut. |

Fill in step 5 with your decision. Even if you choose to do things as you have been doing them, it is now your own decision. It is now a "want," not a "should."

▷ **Step 5:** I've decided to _____

_____

_____

_____

_____

THE LONG METHOD OF CHANGING YOUR VALUES

If you still feel guilty after looking at a "should" that you sense you need to change, use the long method.

Let's take the value of selflessness. Suppose that you were taught that it is wrong to take care of yourself first—that you should take care of other people's needs before your own. Now you wonder whether that is why you feel resentment toward other people.

To determine whether you want to continue to believe this, answer the following questions:

1. Who did I learn my belief from in the first place? Maybe you find yourself thinking about how your mother always put everyone else first and told you that a good parent and spouse always does this.

2. Did I learn my belief because I was afraid not to or because I wanted someone's approval? (Notice who comes to mind as you think about this question.) Maybe you felt afraid of letting your mother down if you didn't do things the way she did, or feared your father's disapproval. Perhaps you heard praise about how well you took care of someone else's needs.

3. What new information do I have to consider that may change my original viewpoint? You've begun to notice that you have a lot of resentment toward your husband and children. You always put their needs first and rarely get what you want. You also remember how much better you felt about your family after you'd been away for a weekend vacation with two friends where you got to do what you really wanted to do.

4. What are some of the side effects or costs of your old belief? Resentment, headaches, and tears can be some side effects of resentment. Irritability, overeating or drinking too much, and depression are other common side effects. At this point maybe you suddenly remember that your mother would take to her bed for several days with a headache every six months or so.

5. What new feelings do you have about your old "should"? Maybe you begin to think that being selfless really doesn't work, that you just end up being upset with other people. Maybe you decide selflessness isn't worth the cost.

CONSIDER ALL THE ALTERNATIVES
↓

THEN DECIDE FOR YOURSELF
↓   ↓

I choose to keep the same value   I choose to change the way I feel
I had when I was young.   about taking care of myself.
                                                  ↓

                                           Have empathy for the former
                                           you who had a different belief.
                                           Under no circumstances should
                                           you put that former you down.
                                           You did the best you could at the
                                           time. You do not need to feel
                                           embarrassed about the younger
                                           you who held a different belief.
                                           That was you then and not you
                                           now. Visualize the former you.
                                           Reach out and give the former
                                           you a big hug.
                                                  ↓

                                           Next, say goodbye to your
                                           former belief.
                                                  ↓

Now the value is your own. It be-   Now, reach out in your imagina-
longs to you because you choose it.   tion to the new belief in the pres-
                                           ent time. Make a commitment
                                           to follow the belief you've found.
                                           As you visualize yourself, extend
                                           a hand and welcome the new
                                           commitment.

↓   ↓

NOW YOUR VALUE IS YOURS.

It doesn't matter what you decide. Your values are your business. What matters is that **you** choose them. It is important that you are conscious of what you believe and why you believe it. Then you can act accordingly, free of guilt and resentment.

▶ Stress Reduction

Stress is a part of everyone's life. It can create physical and emotional problems and symptoms. It can also serve as a reminder that you are simply trying to do something that doesn't fit you. Stress occurs when you get off the path that is growth producing for you. Learning to recognize and handle stress is critical to your well being.

Answer the following questions.

How frequently do you feel stress?

_____ daily   _____ sometimes   _____ rarely

Do you get physically sick frequently?

_____ yes   _____ no

Do you get emotionally upset frequently?

_____ yes   _____ no

Do you get angry a lot?

_____ yes   _____ no

Do you cry a lot?

_____ yes   _____ no

Are you tense or nervous much of the time?

_____ yes   _____ no

Do you have trouble sleeping or have a hard time relaxing?

_____ yes   _____ no

Recognizing the signs that may indicate you are under stress is a step in learning to handle it. The more "yes" responses you have to these questions, the more likely you are to be experiencing stress in your life. To determine the sources of the stress, continue to the next section.

SOURCES OF STRESS

Stress is the result of demands that are being made on us by people, situations, or change in our lives.

Answer the following questions.

Are there a lot of people in your life taking from you, making demands on you, or expecting things from you?

_____ yes   _____ no

List the people and their demands or needs.

Names   Their demands/needs

_____   _____

_____   _____

_____   _____

_____   _____

_____   _____

WHO CREATES STRESS

To help you gain clarity about the people who have an effect on your life, fill in the following chart.

▷ **Step 1:** Place the names of five key people who affect your life on the lines under "Name." It is possible that one or more of the people who influence you are dead. Include them if they still greatly affect your life.

Name   plus or minus sign

_____   _____

_____   _____

_____   _____

_____   _____

_____   _____

▷ **Step 2:** Put "deceased" in front of the name of anyone deceased.

75

▷ **Step 3:** Put a plus (+) or minus (–) sign on the line after each name. A plus indicates that you get as much or more from being around the person than you give. A minus indicates you spend more time and energy being with the person than you get back.

▷ **Step 4:** Add up the total number of pluses.

▷ **Step 5:** Add up the total number of minuses.

You need to have at least as many pluses as you do minuses to keep from being drained. Decide which of the relationships marked with a minus sign you want to keep even though the situation is draining. An example might be a new baby in the home. Though it is draining, it is also a valuable part of your life and you are committed to it.

▷ **Step 6:** List the minuses that you want to keep.

Name _____

Type of drain on you _____

_____

Potential duration of the drain _____

_____

Assistance you can get to help you with this person

Idea 1_____

_____

Idea 2_____

_____

Idea 3_____

_____

The goal is to reduce either the number of people who cause you stress or the effects of the stress caused by them. After trying the ideas listed above, reevaluate the amount of stress you experience in relation to the people in your life. Keep working on getting a positive balance in your life.

SITUATIONS THAT CAUSE STRESS

Stress is also the result of things changing in our lives. The changes can be the result of normal transitions such as growing up, births, marriages, starting or finishing school, and retirement. Or they can be due to losses or additions to your life such as job loss, moving, loss of loved ones, acquisition of a new job, getting a new minister at your religious institution, getting a new boss at work, or adding a new resident to your living quarters.

WHAT CREATES STRESS

To determine what is changing in your life, answer the following questions.

What life transitions have you undergone in the last year?

_____

_____

_____

_____

_____

What life transitions has a family member undergone in the last year? List the person's name followed by the type of change.

_____

_____

_____

_____

_____

When there are many changes to your life or the lives of those to whom you are closely committed, considerable stress results. This is not to say that change is bad. You must take steps, however, to reduce the effects of the change so you can avoid the damage stress can cause to you physically and psychologically. Here are some steps you can take.

▷ **Step 1:** Acknowledge the need to do something about the stress in your life.

▷ **Step 2:** Give yourself permission to ask for help. You may ask for help to divide up chores. Or you may pay someone to assist you with little daily jobs such as housekeeping or filing. Let others do the driving, ask for someone else to make decisions such as where to go for dinner, or ask your spouse to take over the bookkeeping until you feel less stressed.

Say, "I give myself permission to ask for help."

▷ **Step 3:** Be willing to ask for emotional support from others. Rather than volunteering to assist another person, ask to be reassured and nurtured. You may say, "Tell me everything will be all right again," or "Let me know I'm still okay." Be sure to give yourself permission to cry, withdraw temporarily, or take time to do nothing at all. Playing, hiking, or just sunning on a beach can give you the emotional renewal you need.

▷ **Step 4:** Do not begin new projects or press yourself to be creative when you're under a lot of stress.

Say, "I give myself permission to only do what I want to do. I will not press myself to be productive."

What additions to your life have you experienced in the last year?

_____

_____

_____

_____

_____

_____

What losses have you experienced in the last year? Include dreams and opportunities that you feel you have lost.

_____

_____

_____

_____

_____

_____

Anytime you experience additions or losses in your life, you can expect to go through a period of grieving. The old familiar way of life gives way to the new, which is unknown. Most people experience stress and a sense of loss at a time like this. Separation from people and things that are familiar causes a similar grief that needs your attention. (See the section on stages of grief.)

HANDLING ADDITIONS AND LOSSES IN YOUR LIFE

▷ **Step 1:** Acknowledge the change.
▷ **Step 2:** Ask yourself how you feel.

Write how you feel. _____

_____

_____

_____

_____

▷ **Step 3:** Let yourself experience and express the feelings you have at this time. All feelings are equally valid and deserve expression. It is often helpful to ask another person to help you by being a listener.

▷ **Step 4:** Give yourself plenty of time to adjust to the change.

▷ **Step 5:** Do not push yourself to start new things or return to an old schedule of activity or responsibility.

▷ **Step 6:** Consider whether you want to return to old ways or whether you wish to alter your life based on the change.

▷ **Step 7:** In time, accept the change and look at the advantages of having experienced it.

▶ Handling Stress

Ask yourself the following questions.

Do you use drugs or alcohol to relax?

_____ yes   _____ no

Do you use food, shopping, or work to help you feel comfortable?

_____ yes   _____ no

Do you feel better after you have done something thrilling or taken a risk?

_____ yes   _____ no

Does sex help you relax?

_____ yes   _____ no

Answering "yes" to any of these questions means you are trying to cover up your feelings of stress so you don't have to feel them. This is dangerous and easily leads to addiction. Learn new ways to deal with stress. You deserve it.

There are many ways you can handle the results of stressful situations and people. Here are some simple skills that you can use to overcome the effects of stress in your life.

ENVIRONMENTAL MANIPULATION

▷ **Step 1:** Make a list of projects you want to complete and the goals that you want to achieve.

_____   _____

_____   _____

_____   _____

_____   _____

_____   _____

▷ **Step 2:** Now, set priorities. Make four categories.
Category 1: Very important/urgent
Category 2: Quite important
Category 3: Moderately important
Category 4: Can wait/the bottom of the list

▷ **Step 3:** Score each of the twelve items above with a 1, 2, 3, or 4.

▷ **Step 4:** Now rewrite the list of your goals and projects.

Category 1. _____

_____

_____

_____

Category 2. _____

_____

_____

_____

Category 3. _____

_____

_____

_____

Category 4. _____

_____

_____

_____

▷ **Step 5:** Now choose only one item from the first category. I choose_____

_____

▷ **Step 6:** In order to complete the one project, I need to get _____

_____

or I need to ask someone to help me. I choose _____

_____

▷ **Step 7:** Do not try to do any more than the one project. Give yourself permission to finish it before starting another one. Do stress reducing activities before starting another one.

Cutting down on the amount of work you press yourself to do will help you reduce the amount of stress you are under.

BREATHING EXERCISE

One of the most common ways to reduce stress is to breath properly. Learn at least one breathing technique. In addition, be sure to remember to take a few deep breaths regularly.

Deep breathing:
    While stopped in your car at a light, breath deeply and fully for five breaths.
    Right now, inhale deeply, hold your breath to the count of four and exhale to the count of two.
    Stand up at your desk at work. Inhale through your nose and gently exhale through your mouth.
Slow breathing:
    Take a gentle walk and pay attention to your breathing. Breath rhythmically, in and out, in and out. Do not force your breath or hold it. Instead, flow with your breath.

Pay attention to your breathing while doing any kind of relaxation exercises. Make your breathing even and unforced.

RELAXATION EXERCISES

Taking time to relax weary muscles, a tired brain, or drained emotions will ensure a reduction in stress. If you are under stress, you may have had the experience of being too tired to go to sleep. Or you may have fallen into a deep sleep only to awaken with tension still in your muscles. To avoid this, you may need to take an active approach to relaxation.

EXERCISE ONE

▷ **Step 1:** Remove glasses, contacts, and jewelry.

81

▷ **Step 2:** Wearing loose-fitting clothing and lie down on a comfortable surface.

▷ **Step 3:** Starting at the top of your head, wrinkle your brow upwards, holding the pressure for a count of five.

▷ **Step 4:** Release the pressure.

▷ **Step 5:** Tightly close your eyes, holding them shut for a count of five. Release.

▷ **Step 6:** Repeat in the same manner each of the following:

  ▷ Stretch your mouth open as wide as it will go.
  ▷ Turn your head to the far right.
  ▷ Turn your head to the far left.
  ▷ Pull your head forward, touching your chin to your chest.
  ▷ Tip your head back as far as it will go. Remember to hold the body part tightly in the position for a count of five.
  ▷ Clench your right fist and forearm.
  ▷ Clench your left fist and forearm.
  ▷ Tighten your right upper arm.
  ▷ Tighten your left upper arm.
  ▷ Turn your torso to the right, twisting at your waist.
  ▷ Turn your torso to the left, twisting at your waist.
  ▷ Press your shoulder blades together tightly.
  ▷ Encircle yourself across the front with a hug.
  ▷ Tighten your right thigh.
  ▷ Tighten your left thigh.
  ▷ Tighten your right leg below the knee.
  ▷ Tighten your left leg below the knee.
  ▷ Flex your toes upward toward the front of your leg.
  ▷ Point your toes downwards away from your head.

▷ **Step 7:** When you have finished all the stretches, mentally check throughout your body for any places that seem tense.

▷ **Step 8:** Go back and again tighten that area, holding the pressure for a count of five. Then release.

EXERCISE TWO

Jump on a trampoline, jog, run, walk swiftly, dance, or do any form of repetitive exercise that pleases you. Do not force yourself to do some exercise someone else likes unless it feels good to you. Everyone's body is different and deserves to be treated individually.

ARTISTIC OUTLETS

There are all kinds of ways to reduce stress using arts and crafts. If you don't know what you like to do, try a number of things.

▷ **Step 1:** Consider different arts and crafts you can explore: working with clay, painting (ask your local craft store about the various media for painting), sculpture, photography, flower arranging, and many more.

▷ **Step 2:** Visit an arts and crafts store or show to look at materials and finished projects.

▷ **Step 3:** Give yourself permission to experiment with different media. Do not invest a lot of money initially until you have sampled what's available.

▷ **Step 4:** Let yourself experiment on your own if you prefer. If you would rather take some lessons fine, do so, but do not feel pressured.

▷ **Step 5:** After you have settled on one or two different processes that you enjoy, check to be sure you are *not working* at the activity. **Remember, the purpose is relaxation!**

If you do know what you like to do in the artistic area, do it. You may need to carve out the time, but do that.

Write, "I agree to make the time I need to enjoy my art work."

_____

_____

WATER ACTIVITY

Whether you passively enjoy it or actively use it, water provides one of the most time-honored ways in which to relax. Try the following and decide which you like the best.

1. Take a bath with lots of water. Add bubbles if you like. Make the water the temperature you prefer.
2. Take a shower and let it run over your head. Give yourself permission to stay in it for as long as you like. (Warn others in the household that you may use up all the hot water!)
3. Go swimming.
4. Go fishing, with or without a pole. No fussing that you don't catch anything. Remember the purpose.
5. Go boating. To make this a relaxation opportunity, you need to let the boat drift.
6. Sit by running water.
7. Listen to a fountain or a brook.
8. Wade in a stream or other body of water.
9. Go beach walking.

Check the water activities that appeal to you.
Have a wonderful time!

ELECTRONIC RELAXATION

Modern technology has introduced several appliances that allow people with ADD to relax. These include the following:

> Television
>
> Video games
>
> Computers—both games and other activities such as programming, spread sheets, and computer aided design.

A word of warning is necessary, however. It is possible to become addicted to some of these activities, playing them for hours on end. If you are prone to this, here's a tip. Set a timer for the length of time you are willing to spend on the activity. Stop it when the timer goes off. If you cannot stop once you've started, then it is not wise to use these as ways to take a break.

I choose to use the following electronic activity to relax.

Write the name here _____

I am able to stop the activity in an allotted time.

_____ yes   _____ no

I will let myself take breaks that are _____ minutes long.

RELAXATION IN NATURE

Many people with ADD find a great deal of solace by spending time outdoors. This can include passive activities such as

1. lying on your back in the park. Notice the clouds. Do you see shapes in them? Draw a picture or tell a story about what you see.
2. looking at the undersides of the leaves of a tree. Do you see the leaves dancing? Try visualizing a ballet with the individual leaves representing ballerinas.

You may or may not decide to study your surroundings while you walk. Since you are doing this for the purposes of relaxation, don't push yourself. Some people like to listen to a tape player while outside. Do you?

Walking in the country will often improve your mental attitude and make you feel better. You judge the pace you want to set. You do not need to try to push yourself. *Remember, this exercise is for the purpose of relaxation.*

Finally, there are strenuous ways to enjoy the outdoors. Try the following, if they sound interesting:

1. Backpacking.
2. Hiking.
3. Mountain climbing.

PHYSICAL EXERCISE

Physical exercise is a good way for many people to relax. It, too, can be energetic or low-key. You make the decision about what is right for you.

Check or fill in the following blanks.

I would like to play a sport.

_____ yes _____ no

I would like to play_____

_____

_____

As you list the sports that interest you, make a note to check into the availability of amateur games in your area.

I like running.

_____ yes _____ no

I will commit to run on a regular basis.

_____ yes _____ no

I plan to begin running _____ miles per day.

I will run _____ days per week.

I like to dance.

_____ yes _____ no

The kind of music that I like to dance to is _____

_____

_____

I am making a commitment right now to find some places in which I can enjoy my love for dancing. Write them down here as you find out about them. (Be sure to consider programs offered through city parks and recreation departments, ethnic and folk dancing clubs, and free lessons offered on off-nights in some clubs.)

_____

_____

_____

_____

If a partner is required, think about who you might like to take. Fill in the name of the person below. (Remember, asking a friend to go dancing does not necessarily mean you are starting to date the person.)

I'm thinking of asking _____

or _____

Have fun, get good exercise, and feel relaxed afterwards.

MUSIC FOR RELAXATION

Often people with ADD like music. Do not forget, however, that the kind of music you listen to can affect your mood. So if the purpose of listening is to relax, be sure to choose appropriate pieces. Become aware of how different music makes you feel. Then you will learn what is good for you at a given time.

Fill in the following blanks.

I have discovered that I like _____

_____

best for relaxing.

It makes me feel _____

_____

I also like to relax listening to _____

_____

It makes me feel _____

_____

Enjoy! What a nice way to be kind to yourself.

MOVIES

Many people with ADD are movie buffs. Ask yourself:

Do I go to the movies at least once a week?

_____ yes   _____ no

Do I frequently see the same movie more than once?

_____ yes   _____ no

Do I know the actors and actresses and their parts by heart?

_____ yes   _____ no

Do I feel better after I've gone to a movie?

_____ yes   _____ no

You've found a wonderful way to relax if you are an avid movie goer. However, a word of caution. If you're in a committed relationship, do not insist that the other accompany you as often as you would like to go. If the person likes movies as much as you, there probably is no problem. But if not, be sure to try other things that you both may find you like.

MEDITATION AND GUIDED IMAGERY

The development of some form of meditation skills is very helpful to people who have ADD. It doesn't matter whether you choose an active, imaginative type of guided imagery or a quiet, solitary way to become calm. You will know what feels right for you. No one way is better than any other way.

QUIET MEDITATION

▷ **Step 1:** Sit in a quiet place.
▷ **Step 2:** Sweep the thoughts of the day out of your mind. You may wish to mentally put them in a safe place, telling yourself that you will return to them at _____. (Insert the time so your emotions know you are committed.)
▷ **Step 3:** Similarly release all emotions with the same commitment to return to them later.
▷ **Step 4:** Sweep any residual thoughts or feelings out from the center of your mind onto the fringes. Release them.
▷ **Step 5:** Deepen the level of your meditation by moving into the core of your mind that is now blank.
▷ **Step 6:** Check your breathing to be sure it is regular.
▷ **Step 7:** Maintain this level of concentrated meditation for as long as you can, which in the beginning may only be a few minutes.

You can extend the time as you become more adept. You may also find that you benefit from a meditation class.

If the completely quiet meditation does not work for you or doesn't feel good, you may wish to try the following.

1. Add music.
2. Use a repetitive saying such as: "Ommmmm" or "Yes, yes."
3. Hum or sing.
4. Say a prayer.

Check any of the methods that work for you. Become aware of your breathing. Enjoy your meditation.

Finally, you may wish to use guided imagery. In this form, someone leads you on a guided journey. You may wish to join a class or use a pre-recorded tape. Guided imagery

1. Leads you to a place of serenity, such as a beach or the mountains.
2. It describes what is there using soothing terms.
3. It suggests that you feel relaxed, peaceful, and calm.
4. It finishes by guiding you back to the present time and place.

You can even record your own tape with a journey of your choosing. Following is an example.

"As you shut your eyes, imagine that you are in the pine trees on top of a peaceful mountain. The skies are soft blue. Every once in a while, puffy clouds drift lazily by. You can feel yourself walking freely in the forest. Your muscles are relaxing, your head is becoming clear, and your emotions are experiencing calm."

"As your feet touch the forest floor, you notice a slight shifting of your weight as each foot slides smoothly over the pine needles. There is a slight crunching sound underfoot. The needles and the pine cones respond to your movement. They invite you to lie down on them. As you do you feel the smooth, light touch of a mountain breeze caress your cheek. The mountain seems to be breathing with the wind as you become aware of your own breathing. And with every breath that you inhale, you experience calmness and peace. With every breath that you exhale, you know relaxation and a reduction of tension. You feel wonderful."

"A little squirrel runs up the tree trunk near you, swings into the next tree, and finds a friend to play with. Clouds drift lazily by, creating pictures in the sky. As you continue to relax and enjoy yourself, you notice a deer move toward you. It is not the least bit afraid of you. For your part, you are pleased, feeling the soft pleasure of experiencing something unusual and special. And you know that you, too, are special. You are a priceless delight of God. The angels rejoice in your existence. You are a gem of the earth, relaxing and recuperating in a magical forest on the mountain."

This guided imagery can be extended indefinitely. Ten to twenty minutes is plenty to give you the restoration you need.

No one way of meditating or relaxing is better than another. Each is only different from the other. *Remember, no judgments, just pleasure.*

It is important that anyone with ADD learn several ways to reduce stress and use them regularly. A commitment to do so is important, so I am going to ask you to make one now.

I commit to practice some form of stress reduction daily.

I choose the following ways: _____

_____

_____

Feel free to change or vary them any time you want but remember this is an important part of your training program. You deserve to have a low level of stress and enjoy a healthy, happy life.

► ► ►

► Organization and ADD

With high-tech society all around us, organization in daily living has become crucial. However, many people with ADD have a great deal of difficulty getting or keeping themselves organized. Do you experience this difficulty? Answer the following questions.

Do you feel like a failure because you don't know how to organize?

_____ yes _____ no

Do you spend more time looking for things than finding them?

_____ yes _____ no

Are you at a loss when it comes to setting priorities?

_____ yes _____ no

Do you have a way to find things but feel it is not the *right* way?

_____ yes _____ no

89

Are you surrounded by piles of papers?

_____ yes   _____ no

Is your home, car, or workspace chronically untidy?

_____ yes   _____ no

Is it impossible for you to keep track of time?

_____ yes   _____ no

"Yes" responses to these questions indicate either that you have a problem with organization or believe you have a problem. First determine whether you really have a problem or not.

Can you find what you need in your home or office even though they appear disorganized?

_____ yes   _____ no

Can you get a job done under pressure?

_____ yes   _____ no

Are you an effective problem solver if you are left to do it in your own way?

_____ yes   _____ no

Have you lost confidence in your way of accomplishing things?

_____ yes   _____ no

There is a big difference between actually having a problem with organization and *believing* you have one. Realize that

 ▷ the way you reach your goal is your business.
 ▷ completing a project in your own way is just fine.
 ▷ getting a job done is important. How you get it done is not.

PERMISSION TO ORGANIZE THE WAY YOU WANT

There is *no right way* to accomplish a task, though some people believe there is. But that is only a belief. Often children are trained to think they *should* do something in a particular way.

But, really, the particular way is only right for the person speaking.

If you have a way of proceeding with a task that gets the job done, stick with it.

Say, "I give myself permission to work in the way that fits me."

Write, "I give myself permission to organize in the way that fits me even if it doesn't seem organized to others."

Write it here. _____

_____

_____

If a boss or someone else criticizes the way you get the job done, ask which is more important; getting the job done well or appearing organized.

PERFECTIONISM AND ORGANIZATION

Another obstacle to accomplishing tasks effectively is perfectionism. You know this is a problem if you answer "yes" to many of the following questions.

Do you spend so much time organizing that there is no time left to accomplish the task at hand?

_____ yes _____ no

Do you continue to work and rework and redo a task, so much so that you don't complete it on time or at all?

_____ yes _____ no

Do you put off starting a task because you just know you will not be able to complete it perfectly?

_____ yes _____ no

Do you become extremely anxious about doing a task just right?

_____ yes _____ no

There are two reasons for perfectionistic behavior.

▷ One stems from the person's biochemistry.
▷ One is learned.

It is important to differentiate between these two.

Biochemically based perfectionism can be and needs to be treated with medication. If this fits you, it is completely unfair and inhumane to expect yourself to keep trying to do what is beyond you. It is an obsessive-compulsive disorder that can be diagnosed by a mental health professional or physician.

Learned perfectionism is a habit that began as an attempt to get things just right to avoid negative consequences such as scoldings. It can be unlearned when it is safe to do things in your own way without fear of outside reactions.

To correct learned perfectionism, you must give yourself permission to be in charge of the way you do things.

▷ **Step 1:** Decide how much time you want to put in on a given project.

▷ **Step 2:** Assess the audience that will receive or use your project. What are their requirements? Consider using a rating scale made up of percentages such as:

25% perfect   50   75   85   90   95   100

▷ **Step 3:** You may wish to ask the boss or a partner what that person would like.

▷ **Step 4:** Realize a quality job can be done without trying to reach perfection.

▷ **Step 5:** Set a time limit on the project and simply stop when you reach that time.

▷ **Step 6:** Lay out a standard for yourself that allows for a finite amount of correction and refinement. For example, the examples listed in this workbook are representative of the infinite number of possible examples. However, listing many more would make both the writing and reading processes too long. In addition, the fine rewriting and editing could go on indefinitely but would yield decreasing results in terms of readability and would not be worth the time and energy.

▷ **Step 7:** Say, "I give myself permission to do a reasonably good job on the project or assignment."

▷ **Step 8:** Write it. _____

_____

_____

▷ **Step 9:** Follow through on the project and congratulate your-self on a job reasonably well done.

▶ Help with Organization

When you do need help with organization in order to accom-plish the task, there are many things you can do. Your first decision is whether you want assistance with the job or want to do it alone.

▷ Do you want help with the job?
▷ Would you like the job done entirely by someone else?
▷ Do you want to do the job yourself?

DO YOU WANT TO DO YOUR OWN ORGANIZATION?

In order to decide whether you want to do your own organiza-tion, you need to be clear about your skills. But before you can do this, you also must take a look at your beliefs about organi-zation. Here are some guidelines for assessing your skills and beliefs.

▷ **Step 1:** Think about a time when you completed a project. When making your choice, be sure to consider pro-jects that you did easily or wanted to do.

▷ **Step 2:** Do you immediately think or hear dialogue in your mind about how disorderly your approach to doing the project was?

_____ yes _____ no

Do you recall being chastised for leaving it until the last minute?

_____ yes _____ no

Were you teased or even criticized because your desk was messy?

_____ yes _____ no

▷ **Step 3:** Make a note of who told you that your way of approaching the project was not the right way to do it.

Write that name here _____

93

▷ **Step 4:** In reality, did your method of organization work for you to get the job done?

_____ yes _____ no

▷ **Step 5:** Next, look at how much effort it took you to complete the project.

▷ **Step 6:** Are you willing to expend that much energy in order to do your own organization?

▷ **Step 7:** Now decide whether you want to make the effort to do your own organization or would like to look at other options.

Complete: I choose to _____

_____

_____

DO YOU WANT HELP WITH ORGANIZATION?

There are several ways to get assistance with organization.

▷ Teamwork
▷ Make trades
    Exchange services
    Pay money

TEAMWORK

You may find that engaging in team projects suits your purposes well. Using this format, you join forces with one or more people who want to produce the same results you do. The following steps can prove helpful to you.

▷ **Step 1:** When you develop an interest in a project, talk about it. You will tend to discover other people who also are interested. In talking with them you may discover that they have different skills than you have.

▷ **Step 2:** Consider the idea of joining forces. Don't push the idea; just offer it as a possibility. Comfortable, mutually rewarding partnerships come together easily.

▷ **Step 3:** Honestly share the skills you have to offer with the other people and become aware of what they have to offer. All of you together can decide whether you have a full complement of skills that will allow for the successful completion of the project. As a group you may become aware of specific skill needs that are not present and so seek them out.

▷ **Step 4:** Decide within yourself whether your needs can be met by joining forces with these people. The joining can be formal or informal. If you do decide you want to work as a team, let the others know. If you decide you do not want to engage in teamwork, let the others know also so that they can find someone else if they wish to continue.

MAKING TRADES

There is still one more option available to you besides going it alone or becoming a member of a team. You can make trades with people. You can

> ▷ exchange services
> ▷ exchange money

The Exchange of Services: Make a of list services you can exchange for help from another person. You may be a whiz with auto mechanics or gardening. Possibly you would be willing to keep a friend's kids for a weekend in exchange for her organizing of your files.

I can trade the following:

_____	_____
_____	_____
_____	_____
_____	_____
_____	_____

Now list what organizational tasks you need done. Besides your files, desk, closets, and bookkeeping, you may need the development of a checklist in relation to a specific project. An example might be the need for a list of steps to follow in order to get ready for a dinner party for your boss. Or, you might want a series of items purchased for a trip abroad.

I need the following done:

_____	_____
_____	_____
_____	_____
_____	_____
_____	_____

The Exchange of Money: There are times it's best to simply hire a job out. Paying someone to clean your house or organize your closets may be one of the wisest uses you've ever made of your money. Here are some guidelines to accomplish this exchange.

▷ **Step 1:** Give yourself permission to hire a job out.

▷ **Step 2:** If you run into resistance or begin to feel guilty or that you shouldn't pay someone else to do *your* job, ask yourself why. Who did you learn your belief from? Were you taught that a woman's place is in the home and that home must be neatly kept by you? Or did you watch the men in your family change the oil in their cars and think it was the manly thing to do?

▷ **Step 3:** Be willing to either cut back in another area of your budget to pay for the service or do extra work in order to make the extra money needed.

▷ **Step 4:** Enjoy the freedom you've gained by making a monetary trade. Congratulate yourself.

Caution: When you hire work done, pay attention to

▷ the way in which you give the assignment.

▷ the way in which you monitor the progress of the work.

Especially when you feel guilty or insecure, you are likely to have problems with making clear assignments and keeping track of progress.

WAYS IN WHICH ASSIGNMENTS ARE MADE

A Dictaphone can be a valuable tool. You may want to keep one in your pocket or purse.

▷ **Step 1:** Every time you think of something that needs to be done on a project, record it.

▷ **Step 2:** Turn the recorder over to a transcriber who will take the assignments off and order them with regard to importance and timeliness.

▷ **Step 3:** The same person can implement the assignments or turn them over to another person who will do the job.

▷ **Step 4:** You need to be given back a checklist with the date of completion of each item noted.

Written lists fit some people better.

▷ **Step 1:** Note assignments that need to be accomplished. The items do not need to be in order. Neither do they need to be in list form.

▷ **Step 2:** Have the person helping you make an orderly list, checking with you to set priorities. If you wish, ask for a copy of it.

▷ **Step 3:** Be sure each assignment has a due date attached to it. Make a note on your calendar to check about completion. Also ask that a reporting be made to you by a specific date.

MONITORING ASSIGNMENTS

Do not hesitate to have another person monitor the completion of the assignments for you. It is a good idea to stay in touch with that person, however, and regularly get feedback with regard to the progress of the work.

Consider the way in which you want the feedback given.

Do you want a written report?

_____ yes   _____ no

If so, do you want an outline of results or a fairly complete, detailed report of accomplishments?

I want _____

_____

Would you like a verbal report?

_____ yes   _____ no

Do you want it followed up with a written summary?

Immediately mark your calendar or datebook with bold markings to cue you to check on any incomplete results.

DO-IT-YOURSELF ORGANIZATION

Even when some aspects of organization in your life can be transferred to other people, there will remain some things that you need to do for yourself. To make that job easier, here are some pointers.

Typical areas that make trouble for people with ADD include

▷ time management
▷ keeping track of things
▷ long-term projects
▷ setting priorities
▷ changing your mind and other areas of flexibility

Each of these areas can cause a lot of trouble in your life. But you can also learn to get control of each of these areas. Tackle them one at a time and become the successful person you were always meant to be.

TIME MANAGEMENT

For people with ADD, dealing with time can be hard.

> ▷ You may find it difficult to keep track of time.
> ▷ You may become completely absorbed in whatever you are doing, not realizing that time is passing.
> ▷ You may struggle with using time in your best interest; for example, rushing when you don't need to and letting your attention wander when you need to focus.

If you have trouble keeping track of time, use whatever aids you need to help yourself.

Mechanical Aids: Alarms and timers that intrude into your senses often help. These can be auditory, visual, or kinesthetic.

Auditory aids include alarm clocks that ring or buzz. Watches set to go off when it is time to take medication can help a lot. Don't forget the metronome to help with pacing an activity. Originally designed for use by musicians to assist with keeping the beat, it can help a person find his rhythm in any activity.

Visual aids include the three-minute egg timer to keep track of how much has been accomplished in what length of time. Digital timers can be set for a specific length of time. They then can be observed with regard to the amount of time left to complete a task. This can provide the motivation to keep "on task." Digital clocks, too, seem to benefit people with ADD. They are easy to read, and the way they report time seems to provide a structure that is beneficial to people with ADD.

Kinesthetic aids set up a vibration that will cue you. Placed in your pocket, such an aid will begin to vibrate at the time you set it. Thus you have a reminder to alert you to a need for a change in activity. Others vibrate at intervals, thus nudging you to pay attention.

People Aids: Don't hesitate to ask people to help you stay on task. Many a partnership can benefit both people. This works especially well when you have a tendency to overfocus on an activity.

> ▷ **Step 1:** Ask someone to be your partner.
> ▷ **Step 2:** Give that person permission to remind you about time.

98

▷ **Step 3:** Vow to yourself that you will stop when the person tells you time is up. Absolutely no fudging is allowed.

▷ **Step 4:** Thank the person for doing so.

▷ **Step 5:** Congratulate yourself.

Say to yourself, "I can learn to manage time with help."

Write about the first time you manage time effectively using any aid you wish. _____

_____

_____

REWARDS AND TIME MANAGEMENT

It is important to reward yourself for concentrating on a task, especially one that you are happy about doing. Give yourself a break.

▷ **Step 1:** Make a list of things that can serve as a reward for you. Anything you like to do such as read, watch TV, or talk on the phone can be a reward.

_____ _____

_____ _____

_____ _____

▷ **Step 2:** Set a limit on the time you will spend enjoying your reward. For example, if you are reading a book, you might want to limit yourself to ten pages. (Be careful. One man limited himself to a chapter. It worked as long as the chapters were twenty pages long but you can imagine what happened when he came to one that was seventy pages.)

▷ **Step 3:** You must be absolutely resolved to follow your own rules and guidelines about using your rewards. TV provides a good example. You may watch one thirty minute show. The moment it is over, the TV must be turned off, not down. If any of the next show, even the preview is shown, you are likely to find you've watched the whole show without realizing it.

Support groups for people with ADD will provide you with many opportunities to learn ways to keep track of time. There are also catalogues of devices designed for use by children and adults who have ADD and learning disabilities. Experiment and know that you can improve your ability to manage time.

KEEPING TRACK OF THINGS

Many systems are available to help people keep track of their schedules, projects, inventories, and other needs. You may need to do a bit of experimenting to see what fits you.

Ask yourself the following:

Do you like computers?

_____ yes   _____ no

If you do, there are computerized software packages that can do the trick for you.

Do you like to write and put reminders in boxes and between lines on paper?

_____ yes   _____ no

If you do, you will probably prefer to carry a date book organizer and learn to use it. Do not give up easily if you don't use it effectively at first. It does take practice. Learning to use it can be a good activity for a group of people with ADD to undertake together.

Do you prefer to use a blank sheet of paper to design your own schedule for the day, week, or month?

_____ yes   _____ no

Some people like to draw balloons telling them what to do, just like cartoons. Others like to use colored markers to highlight the activities they want to do.

Do you like to have a special slot, box, or shelf for different projects?

_____ yes   _____ no

If you do, there are plastic organizers, files of all shapes and sizes, and dividers and containers to suit any taste. Before committing to much expense, put some time into looking at what's on the market. Try a small organizational unit to see whether you will actually use it.

If you are a reader, you may like to use tabs and dividers that are marked with subjects and/or colored labels. These may serve to cue you making it easy for you to keep track of your papers and other things.

Do you simply like to have stacks?

_____ yes   _____ no

If you do, stick to your method. The issue is whether you can find things when you want them without spending too much time. Every once in a while you may choose to house clean. But that may only need to get done once or twice a year. The nice thing about this method is that much can be thrown away as no longer timely. It helps in the setting of priorities.

LONG-TERM PROJECTS

The biggest problem that people with ADD have with long-term projects is failing to break them down into manageable bits.

Ask yourself the following:

Do I have trouble knowing where to start a big project?

_____ yes   _____ no

Do many projects seem just too big to manage?

_____ yes   _____ no

Do I have trouble going from one step to another?

_____ yes   _____ no

Do I reward myself for accomplishing little bits of a project?

_____ yes   _____ no

Can I only work on a crisis basis?

_____ yes   _____ no

Do I know how to create the opportunities for little victories so I can get a sense of accomplishment as I pursue a long-term goal?

_____ yes   _____ no

Take a look at your answers and check the ones that you need to work on. To obtain further clarification and gain experience, do the following exercise.

▷ **Step 1:** Choose a project. Pick one that has several steps to it.

▷ **Step 2:** Write a brief description of the project. For example, you may choose to clean off the top of a desk that has gone untouched for years. Or you might need to write a report that is twenty-five pages long.

I choose to work on _____

_____

_____

_____

▷ **Step 3:** Now, ask yourself, "What is the first thing that needs to be done?" If you feel confused or have no idea where to start, you need a plan. There is more than one stage to the development of your plan.

Stage One: On a blank sheet of paper, write as many of the parts or aspects of the project as you are aware of.

The desk project: 1) Sort what I find into groupings labeled, "Have to keep," "Throw away," and "Not sure." 2) Dispose of the various groups. 3) Clean the top of the desk. 4) Set up an organizational method that I can follow.

The twenty-five page report: 1) What is the purpose of the report? 2) What needs to be included in the report? 3) What background information do I need to obtain in order to write it? 4) Do I need research done? 5) Who can do it. 6) What form does the report need to be in? 7) Who will type the report?

Stage Two: Go back over the material you collected in stage one and begin to order it. Ask yourself, "What needs to be done first?" For example, with the desk, you need to sort through the papers first. With the report, you must discover the purpose of the report before you do anything with it.

▷ **Step 4:** Make your plan of attack step by step.

▷ **Step 5:** Number the steps.

▷ **Step 6:** Go back over the steps one at a time to determine if any of them can be broken down further. For example, with the desk you may want to divide the sorting step into two segments: one for loose papers and one for other things. For the report you may want to divide the purpose-discovery segment into two parts: one for asking what your supervisor wants, one considering what you believe or feel should be in the report.

▷ **Step 7:** Consider ways to divide up the project. This could be done in terms of time spent or areas covered. The desk could be divided into four parts with the first part being done the first day. The report could be started with your limiting the amount of time you choose to spend at one sitting. You could also limit yourself by only working on the purpose initially. Then stop and continue the next day or an hour later on the next step, which might be to consider the background material you need to collect. Then stop again.

▷ **Step 8:** You may wish to use the following outline to help you.

Project _____

_____

Check when
completed   Describe steps

_____   1. _____

_____   2. _____

_____   3. _____

_____   4. _____

_____   5. _____

_____   6. _____

_____   7. _____

_____   8. _____

_____   9. _____

_____   10. _____

_____   11. _____

_____   12. _____

_____   13. _____

_____   14. _____

_____   15. _____

_____   16. _____

_____   17. _____

_____   18. _____

_____   19. _____

_____   20. _____

▷ **Step 9:** Be sure to liberally sprinkle rewards for completing segments of your project. They can be anything from a five-minute telephone conversation to a walk to the water cooler. You can tally up your rewards and turn them in on a prize for yourself when the project is over. For example, you might put five dollars in a jar each time you complete a segment. If there are twenty segments, you would earn a hundred dollars when you complete the project and could use that to get something you've been wanting for a while.

▷ **Step 10:** Realize that any project can be made manageable by breaking it down. You no longer need to be afraid that you can't handle long-range projects.

SETTING PRIORITIES

When you are clear with yourself and others about what you are and are not willing to do in relation to a project, you will discover it is simple to set priorities.

When you take your courage in your hands to do what you want to do, you will find it easy to set priorities.

When you see the overview of a project with a clear understanding of the outcome you desire from the project, you will be able to order the steps needed to accomplish the job. In turn, you will be able to set priorities.

Ask yourself the following:

Do I always put off doing what I really love to do and then never get around to it?

_____ yes   _____ no

Do I feel obligated to do things I don't really want to do?

_____ yes   _____ no

Can I give myself permission to let others do what I don't want to do?

_____ yes   _____ no

Am I able to delegate responsibility for the things I do not want to do?

_____ yes   _____ no

Am I honest with myself about what I do and don't want to do?

_____ yes   _____ no

Do I let my heart's desires guide me?

_____ yes   _____ no

Am I able to see the purpose of a project, to get the overview?

._____ yes   _____ no

Do I know what outcome I want from a project?

_____ yes   _____ no

In order to effectively set priorities, you need to follow simple guidelines.

- ▷ Do what you are willing to do.
- ▷ Do not do anything you don't want to do.
- ▷ Do what makes you feel best.
- ▷ Do what your heart desires.
- ▷ Be clear with yourself
- ▷ Be honest with others.
- ▷ Take the entire project into consideration.
- ▷ Know the kind of outcome you wish to receive from the project.

Make a check by each guideline with which you are willing to work.

Keep in mind your vision of what you are and are not willing to do and know that you are capable of setting priorities.

CHANGING YOUR MIND AND OTHER AREAS OF FLEXIBILITY

Getting bogged down because you are no longer interested in a project is not unusual. It is especially hard for someone with ADD to focus on a job that is no longer of interest.

Respond to the following questions to check yourself.

Do I prefer to start projects rather than carry them out?

_____ yes   _____ no

Am I able to purposefully make a decision to stop a project part-way through if I want to?

_____ yes   _____ no

Can I imagine any options other than finishing the project to the end myself or quitting all together?

_____ yes _____ no

All of these questions center around the ideas of flexibility and options. There are healthy ways to change your mind and hurtful and destructive ways to do so.

To change your mind in a healthy manner, follow these guidelines.

> ▷ Be who you are.
> If you are an entrepreneur, then act as one. Don't try to do the whole show yourself. Start projects and get a partner to carry them on.
> ▷ Act honestly on what you feel.
> If you get midway through a project and find your interest flagging, stop. Think. Assess your feelings. Then decide what you want to do. If you decide to finish it, know that you have made the decision.
> ▷ Consider at least three options for every situation you face.
> Rather than thinking only in terms of whether or not to do the project, investigate ways to get the project completed without your having to do it, or do all of it. Talk with other people about options, too.

THE ON-OFF SWITCH

People with ADD generally seem to have difficulty getting started on a project. But once started, they often have an equally difficult time stopping what they are doing. It is as if the phonograph needle gets stuck in one groove and can't make it over into the next one.

What you don't want to do if you have trouble in this area is

> ▷ feel guilty
> ▷ hide your behavior
> ▷ lie
> ▷ isolate yourself from others
> ▷ cease doing things

What you do want to do is

> ▷ recognize the problem
> ▷ be open about the difficulty with yourself and others
> ▷ be honest
> ▷ be firm but kind with yourself about overcoming it
> ▷ ask others to help you overcome the problem
> ▷ practice starting and stopping activities

If you are willing to work with this difficulty, proceed.

▷ **Step 1:** Acknowledge to yourself that you often get stuck starting and stopping activities.

▷ **Step 2:** Commit to yourself that you want to change and can change. Say, "I want to change my behavior. I can change my behavior and become more flexible starting and stopping what I do."

Write it _____

_____

_____

▷ **Step 3:** Ask someone to help you. Often, having someone give you a reminder will begin to modify the "on-off" switch.

▷ **Step 4:** If the person agrees, make a pact that you will practice starting your activity with a reminder from the person.

▷ **Step 5:** Ask for a reminder from the person after a reasonable time to stop has been reached. Decide on this amount of time beforehand.

▷ **Step 6:** After some practice with a helper, you can use other devices to serve as reminders such as a clock alarm. Eventually you will have improved to the point that you will be able to overcome the problem simply by thinking about wanting to stop or start at a certain time.

A variation of the on-off switch problem is the either-or switch. There frequently seems to be little or no middle ground for people with ADD. It is as if there are only two settings, this or that. No third or fourth alternatives seem to be available.

For example, suppose an ADD family wants to go on a vacation. Maybe the parents want to go to the mountains and the kids want to go to the beach. Neither seems willing to give in to the other side, thus giving up on what they want to do. It's either the beach or the mountains. It never occurs to anyone that perhaps the first part of the vacation could be at the beach and the second part could be in the mountains. Or that one year they could go one place and the next go another. Or that the kids could go with the neighbors or grandparents who love to go to the beach while the parents go to the mountains.

Options, option, options!

To work with the either-or difficulty, proceed.

▷ **Step 1:** List at least three solutions to every impasse.

▷ **Step 2:** Practice on small things like where to go out for dinner or what game to play at home. This practice will be transferrable to bigger choices later.

▷ **Step 3:** Congratulate yourselves on a job well done.

As you develop your flexibility, be aware that at first it may feel strange, but after a while you will become more and more skillful. It will get easier and easier.

Say to yourself,

"I can become a flexible person."

"I have many options to get jobs done."

"I can learn to get a project done in my own way, in my own time."

Congratulate yourself!

▶ ▶ ▶

▶ Interpersonal Relations

Getting along with other people can be difficult for anyone, but when you have ADD you can be sure the level of skill needed to accomplish harmony increases. However, you have already learned a lot about staying in control of yourself despite having ADD. Now it's time to proceed to the next step—staying in control of yourself in your relationships.

If this interests you, ask yourself the following:

Do I have trouble getting along with people?

_____ yes   _____ no

Do my relationships often end in a fight that never gets resolved?

_____ yes   _____ no

Is it hard for me to stay in a relationship for more than a short while?

_____ yes   _____ no

Do I often get into relationships with people who harm me?

_____ yes   _____ no

Do I feel bruised from being hurt in relationships?

_____ yes   _____ no

Do I feel misunderstood much of the time?

_____ yes   _____ no

Do I feel guilty much of the time in relationships?

_____ yes   _____ no

Is it hard for me to understand what another person needs?

_____ yes   _____ no

Do I know how to solve problems with others?

_____ yes   _____ no

Is it hard for me to be intimate with someone else?

_____ yes   _____ no

Can I set limits with others?

_____ yes   _____ no

Do I know how to handle someone who makes my life their business?

_____ yes _____ no

Am I being pulled in more than one direction at a time by people I love?

_____ yes _____ no

If you answered "yes" to any of the questions, proceed. It's time for you to learn specific skills that will help you have successful, happy relationships. You deserve them.

► Communication

Communication is the backbone of interpersonal relationships. It is a skill that can be learned any time. You can also relearn poor communication skills any time.

Communication takes place both verbally and nonverbally. Actions speak as loud as words. If you communicate in a healthy, open manner, you

- ▷ say what you mean
- ▷ listen to others
- ▷ respond to others when they speak
- ▷ follow through on what you promise
- ▷ can be counted on to be lovable and livable

CHARACTERISTIC PATTERNS OF COMMUNICATION

Several patterns seem to be characteristic of people with ADD. They include

- ▷ dishonesty
- ▷ the "uh-huh" syndrome discussed earlier
- ▷ overcommitment
- ▷ communicating through your behavior: gestures, looks, posture

DISHONESTY

If this is a problem for you, you probably aren't intentionally dishonest. Dishonesty is motivated by fear. It doesn't mean you are a bad person, just a scared one.

Answer the following questions to check yourself.

Do you tell people what they want to hear rather than disappoint them?

_____ yes   _____ no

Is it possible you gloss over the truth, fearing that the listener will think poorly of you if you share what you really think or feel?

_____ yes   _____ no

Are you able to say "no"?

_____ yes   _____ no

If you answered "yes" to some of these, know that it takes a lot of courage to be truthful. Here are some facts that may make the job easier.

ABOUT HONESTY

Fact 1. Anytime you tell someone what he wants to hear, you are only putting off the inevitable.

Fact 2. The longer you put off telling the truth, the harder it becomes to be honest.

Fact 3. The more time that passes before the person finds out the truth, the harder it is for him to adjust to it.

ABOUT GLOSSING OVER THE TRUTH

Fact 1. Anything you try to hide will pop out when you least expect it.

Fact 2. When it does pop out, it will cause more trouble than it would have initially.

Fact 3. Whitewashing the truth breaks down the trust between two people.

ABOUT FAILING TO SAY "NO"

Fact 1. If you say "yes" when you mean "no," you will create a big problem for everyone involved.

Fact 2. You will end up making others mad at you if you try to please them by saying "yes" when you don't mean it.

Fact 3. You will feel angry at the other person if you say "yes" when you really want to say "no."

To be honest in your communication, you must learn to *tell the truth.* Follow the steps below.

▷ **Step 1:** Make a commitment to learn this skill.

▷ **Step 2:** Tell a friend about your commitment.

▷ **Step 3:** Regularly report to your friend (daily if necessary) about your progress.

▷ **Step 4:** Ask your friend to reinforce you for each success you have in speaking the truth.

▷ **Step 5:** Go back to someone to whom you told a lie.

▷ **Step 6:** Tell the truth and tell *why* you told the lie. Talk about how you felt—your fears and needs.

▷ **Step 7:** Again commit to tell the truth from now on.

▷ **Step 8:** Say, "Thank you for listening."

▷ **Step 9:** Repeat steps 5 through 8 with each person to whom you told a lie.

To be honest in your communication, *tell the whole story.* Allowing yourself to omit parts of a story or to keep secrets breaks down trust between you and other people. Frequently there is a sense that something is missing or not quite right. This leads to speculation that maybe there is something very wrong when really you've only chosen to leave out a little bit of the truth. To correct this problem, follow these steps.

▷ **Step 1:** Go to the person to whom you failed to tell the whole story. Say, "I didn't tell you why I lost my job. I realize you thought there'd been a lay-off and I didn't correct you."

111

▷ **Step 2:** Say *why* you didn't tell the whole truth. For example, "I was afraid you'd get mad at me and not want to see me any more."

▷ **Step 3:** Tell what really happened. "I quit because I got really mad when my boss accused me of not getting all my reports in on time when I had gotten them in on time. Can I help it if his secretary misfiled my reports?"

▷ **Step 4:** Tackle the question of trust. You might say, "I realize it may be hard for you to trust me now, but that's the only time I didn't tell the whole story."

▷ **Step 5:** Give the person permission to take time to rebuild trust in you.

▷ **Step 6:** Apologize. Keep it simple. "I'm sorry. I think I've learned my lesson—painfully."

Do you want to make exceptions to this? Is this for all subjects with all people, or only with close friends? What about events or issues that involve other people's privacy and not just your own? To be honest in your communication, you must *be able to say "no."* Follow these steps.

▷ **Step 1:** Think of some simple thing that you said you'd do but don't really want to do.

▷ **Step 2:** Go to the person involved and say, "I told you I would fix the bathroom sink but I really don't want to."

▷ **Step 3:** Suggest an alternative way to get the job done.

▷ **Step 4:** The next time you are asked to do something that you really don't want to do, say, "No, I really won't be able to do that." If you forget at first to say "no," stop as soon as you realize you don't want to do it and say, "On second thought, I need to say 'no.' I'm sorry if I'm letting you down."

▷ **Step 5:** Know that you are breaking an old habit and congratulate yourself.

You are now ready to see yourself as an honest person. Once you can believe in yourself, you will feel very proud. Gone are the days when you needed to be afraid of disapproval for being dishonest. You can now believe in yourself.

OVERCOMMITMENT

If you know the feeling of not working up to your potential, you may have gotten into the habit of overcommitting to try to prove you really are valuable. Or you may be so excited by being able to work closer to your potential that you want to do *everything*.

Ask yourself the following:

Do I take on more projects than I can complete satisfactorily?

_____ yes _____ no

Even if others tell me I've done a good job, do I feel someone else could have done it better?

_____ yes _____ no

Am I always self-critical about what I accomplish?

_____ yes _____ no

Do I feel insecure?

_____ yes _____ no

Do I feel I've lost a lot of time in my life and want to do it all now?

_____ yes _____ no

Do I believe I need to implement every idea that comes into my head?

_____ yes _____ no

Do I crave the high I feel when I begin something new?

_____ yes _____ no

Overcommitting is

▷ often an attempt to prove that you *can do it all.* Inherent in this attitude is the belief that *you are not valuable.* It means you must continually prove you are valuable.
▷ sometimes the result of feeling you want to make up for lost time.
▷ a desire to experience the feeling of beginning a project. There is a high at the initiation of an activity that can be very addictive. Craving this feeling is not unusual.

To remedy the habit of overcommitting, follow these steps.

▷ **Step 1:** First overcome the cause of your overcommitment. If you feel *insecure about yourself or your performance*

tell yourself,
"I am a valuable person."
"My skills are valuable."
"I believe in myself."

113

then say,
"I can release the old beliefs about my inadequacy."

If you are *trying to make up for lost time*

tell yourself,
"There is plenty of time to do the things that are important."
"I have enough time to do what I want."
"I can pick and choose what I do."
"I am in control of my time."

If you *crave the high of beginning a project*

tell yourself,
"I can feel *wonderful,* too, about completing a project."
"I can *feel* the great feeling I had the last time I began a project. I do not have to start a new one to get the feeling."

▷ **Step 2:** Write down the current projects you are involved with or have been asked to do.

▷ **Step 3:** Divide them into three groups.

Group 1 projects are labeled "I have to do these." You would do these even if you had a million dollars.

Group 2 projects are labeled "I'd like to do these." You want to do these but can skip them, if necessary.

Group 3 projects are labeled "I'd rather not do these." You let yourself be talked into these or think you *should* do them. You would feel relieved to skip these.

▷ **Step 4:** Call the people associated with the third group immediately. Resign, decline, or ask for someone to help you carry the project as you cannot continue. *Do not lie.* Tell the truth, saying you overcommitted, and apologize. Do what you can to help find a replacement. If *absolutely* necessary, complete the project *and* delegate a lot of the jobs. Be honest with others about what the problem is.

▷ **Step 5:** Go over the group 1 list. Set priorities if there is more than one project. Your priorities may be due to interest on your part, resources available, or a time factor associated with the project.

▷ **Step 6:** Make an estimate of how long it will take you to complete the group 1 projects. Include how many hours a day you can reasonably work. Do not forget to make time for family, personal relationships, fun, and body/mind/spirit care. If you have trouble with this step, ask a friend, mentor, or counselor to help you.

▷ **Step 7:** If there is any time left in your schedule, turn to the group 2 project list. Set priorities.

▷ **Step 8:** Choose only as many as will comfortably fit what you can accomplish.

Your job is to stick to these steps. You can do it with a little practice. Then, watch your life improve.

COMMUNICATING THROUGH YOUR BEHAVIOR

Remember, communication is both verbal and nonverbal. And actions speak as loud as words. To maintain happy, healthy interpersonal relations, it is important that your words match your actions. To be liveable, you need to be able to follow-through on what you say. But for people with ADD, this follow-through can be very difficult.

Ask yourself the following:

Do I agree to things but then forget to do them?

_____ yes   _____ no

Do others get angry at me because of my behavior?

_____ yes   _____ no

Have I often *talked* my way out of problem situations?

_____ yes   _____ no

Am I well-meaning but hard to live with?

_____ yes   _____ no

Do I know how to look or act cute in order to get out of tight situations?

_____ yes   _____ no

Any of these behaviors are a sign that your actions and your words need to be more in tune with each other. To accomplish this, you must first learn some facts about communication.

Fact 1. Any words you speak are only as valuable as the actions that support them.

Fact 2. Lack of follow-through will catch up with you sooner or later as others begin to distrust or discount you.

115

Fact 3. You do not deserve to be discounted. You are too valuable for that.

Fact 4. Though ADD contributed to your poor follow-through, you *learned* that it was acceptable to be irresponsible. (Even though your parents or teachers scolded you, they did not insist on follow-through by you.)

Fact 5. Because this is a learned behavior, you can unlearn it.

► Turning Words into Actions

If you would like to learn to match your actions to your words, continue. Then, you can become known as a person "whose word is as good as his deed."

Think of a typical situation where you have said one thing and done another.

Write it here. _____

_____

_____

_____

An example could be saying you were going to file your income tax but not doing it. Or maybe you have an outstanding traffic ticket that you *said* you'd pay. Maybe you agreed to fix the bathroom plumbing—two years ago. Or maybe your office still has stacks of papers all around after you said you'd get to them.

Ask yourself the following:

What was I thinking when I spoke?

Write it here. _____

_____

_____

_____

Did I *intend* to fail to follow through?

_____ yes _____ no

Was I even thinking about following through?

_____ yes _____ no

Who accomplished follow-through for me in the past? My parents, spouse, friend? _____

Is the job still undone?

____ yes ____ no

Now answer the following:

Are you ready to *accomplish* follow-through?

_____ yes _____ no

Are you scared you'll fail?

_____ yes _____ no

If you answered "yes," thanks for being honest. You are courageous. You *can* learn to break the task down into small, manageable segments that *you can accomplish.* You *can* learn to turn your words into action. Say, "I can do it." If you are honestly not scared or apprehensive about taking charge, more power to you. It is time to succeed.

You must go through two stages to get on top of your situation.

Stage One: Train yourself to follow through.
Stage Two: Use your brain to train your mouth to be discriminating in its verbalizations.

Proceed with stage one.

▷ **Step 1:** Begin by doing one thing toward your goal. For example, get the phone number of an accountant to help you with your taxes. Or call the office that handles traffic tickets and find out how much you owe. For the plumbing project decide whether you even *want* to do it. Take *one,* not two, pieces of paper off the first pile by the office door and either throw it away, put it in a box, or ask a friend what to do with it. Complete this step before proceeding.
▷ **Step 2:** Now congratulate yourself because you know you *can* follow through to accomplish what you want.
▷ **Step 3:** Continue breaking the job down to complete the project of your choice. Fill in the following:

Project _____

_____

Steps	Accomplished
_____	_____
_____	_____
_____	_____
_____	_____
_____	_____
_____	_____

▷ **Step 4:** Decide what you want your reward to be when you complete the project.

I want to _____

_____

_____

_____

If the project has a lot of steps or stretches over a long period of time, plan several mini-celebrations along the way.

Mini-celebrations _____

_____

_____

_____

Proceed to stage two.

Use your brain to train your mouth to be discriminating. Though the particular brain chemistry of ADD often leads to speaking before you think, your brain can also use its thinking capabilities to help curb this tendency.

▷ **Step 1:** Begin to listen to yourself as you speak. Your words are important—important enough for you to listen. Do this by spending five minutes with someone you trust. (Pairing off within a group is a great way to accomplish this.) Talk about anything. But every time you speak a sentence, stop and repeat the sentence a second time to your partner. Say, "I said _____." Then go ahead and say the next thing.

▷ **Step 2:** Repeat the exercise but this time use a sensitive topic, one that may have gotten you into trouble recently. Your spouse or parent can probably tell you what this is.

▷ **Step 3:** Next, practice this skill out in the world. Listen to yourself as you go through the day. Are you saying what you want to be saying? Are you willing to translate your words into actions? Make conscious decisions about this.

▷ **Step 4:** Congratulate yourself on a job well done.

▷ **Step 5:** Now take on the more difficult task of applying lesson to situations that are stressful. Practice the steps when you are under stress or are angry.

▷ **Step 6:** When you are under stress, do not say anything initially. Stop, look, and listen. Walk away if necessary to give yourself time to think. Thinking is the key.

▷ **Step 7:** Decide how you want to handle the situation and what you want to say. Proceed.

▷ **Step 8:** Congratulate yourself. You have developed a habit that you can carry with you for the rest of your life.

You have learned a new pattern of communication that will make your interpersonal relations easier and more pleasant. You are now someone who can be counted on to "put your money where your mouth is." Good for you!

▶ Skills for Clear Communication

You first learned to communicate when you were a child. It's now time to check and see whether you have the skills for *clear* communication.

Ask yourself the following questions:

Do I seem to be understood when I communicate?

_____ yes _____ no

Do my needs not get met even though I think I am communicating them to others?

_____ yes _____ no

Do other people sometimes get mad at me when I'm asking them for something?

_____ yes _____ no

Do I know how to negotiate with other people so I can get what I want?

_____ yes _____ no

119

Do I know how to make trades with other people so we each get what we want?

_____ yes   _____ no

The satisfactory answer to each of these questions is dependent upon the clarity of your communication. Often people *think* they are communicating but their communications are not perceived the way they were intended. Here are several skills that will help you become more effective.

- ▷ "I" communications
- ▷ Asking for help
- ▷ Identification and clear communication of needs
- ▷ Cutting a deal
- ▷ Problem-solving joint needs

"I" COMMUNICATIONS

Many times people think they have asked for what they want only to find out that the other person didn't get the message. A typical example:

> You come home from a hard day at the office. You sigh as you enter your home and say, "Wouldn't you like to go out to dinner?" The response back is, "Not really. I thought I'd watch the ball game," or "Not really. My hair isn't fixed." In response, you feel disappointed, maybe angry. Perhaps you think that your loved one doesn't care that you are tired. In all likelihood you get mad and throw a remark back, starting a fight. Or it could be that you walk off, pouting for the rest of the evening.

The problem here can be found on one word. Can you find it? The word is "you." You said, "Wouldn't *you* like to go out to dinner?" instead of *"I would like to go out to dinner."*

Use the word "I" to state clearly what you want: I want, I need, I'd like. *You must say what you want if you are to be heard.*

If this makes you feel uncomfortable, you may wish to do the next section first.

Here are some practice opportunities:

1. Repeat, "I want to go out to dinner."
   "I need to sleep with the fan on."
   "I would prefer you smoke outside."
2. Make up your own.

   "I want_____."

   "I need _____."

   "I would prefer_____."

A word of caution. Do not give a lot of reasons why you want what you want when you want it. You don't need to build a case for why you deserve something you want. Just state your desire.

On the other hand, it is okay to give a simple explanation statement that reflects how you feel. For example, "I'm tired. I want to go out to dinner."

Practice using no more than five words of explanation.

"I feel _____, so

I want to _____."

"I feel _____, so

I'd like to_____."

Good for you!

A second word of caution. When you use the "I" method of communication, you must be prepared to receive a "no" answer. You can try to find out whether there is some way that you and the other person can reach a mutually satisfactory solution.

You might say, "Is there some way that you would be able to get what you need and I can get what I need?" If the person is willing to consider this option, go to the section on negotiation skills in communication. If not, accept the "No" and take care of yourself. Take yourself out to dinner.

ASKING FOR WHAT YOU WANT

When you have been trained to be polite or unselfish, or taught that it is improper to be forthright about your needs, you may have trouble asking for what you want. More than likely you found the previous exercise difficult if not impossible. It's time to give yourself a friendly bit of support and a gentle nudge to become responsible to get your own needs met.

Rather than trying to convince yourself to be responsible for your needs, ask whether you have any of the following difficulties:

Do you feel resentful because others do not appreciate what you do?

_____ yes   _____ no

Do you suffer from a lot of depression that could stem from not getting your needs met?

_____ yes   _____ no

Are there never enough hours in the day so that you can get around to something for yourself?

____ yes   ____ no

Are you the last person on your priority list of obligations?

____ yes   ____ no

Do you feel guilty when you take any time for yourself?

____ yes   ____ no

Do you feel deserving?

____ yes   ____ no

Sooner or later neglecting yourself will catch up with you.

- ▷ You may become physically ill so you have an excuse to be taken care of.
- ▷ Similarly, you may become emotionally drained and *have* to take time off to get your needs met.
- ▷ You may lose control of your life and not understand why you can't *make things happen* any longer.
- ▷ Your self esteem may deteriorate.

You don't need to wait for any of these things to happen. Instead you can take the lead and become responsible for your own needs without hurting others. Keep the focus here on meeting your own needs.

Begin.

- ▷ **Step 1:** Give yourself permission to ask for help. Say to yourself, "I give myself permission to ask for help." Say it three times a day: morning, noon, and at bedtime.

- ▷ **Step 2:** Write it _____

  _____

  Signature_____ Date _____

  Skip to Step 5 if you feel all right with 1 and 2.

- ▷ **Step 3:** If you run into difficulty doing step 1 or 2, ask yourself, "Who expected me to be responsible

  for their feelings and needs?" _____

  _____

How old was I when it started?_____

_____

Who do I now know/live with who expects me to be responsible for them? (Children do not count— though it is important to only do for them what they cannot do for themselves.)

_____

_____

▷ **Step 4:** Either conjure up a mental picture of the person or look at a photograph. Say, "You did not intend to hurt me when you made me responsible for your feelings and comfort, but you did. I didn't feel I had a choice. Now I know differently. I do have a choice."

"I forgive both of us for our roles in this situation."
"I give you back responsibility for yourself."
"I take responsibility for myself."

▷ **Step 5:** Say, "I am now ready to begin to ask for what I need."

▷ **Step 6:** Select something small with which you would like assistance. Maybe it is help with the dishes or getting the car in for service.

▷ **Step 7:** Choose the person you want to ask to help you.

▷ **Step 8:** Go to the person and say, "I wonder if you

would be willing to help me. I need _____

_____

Will you do it?"

▷ **Step 9:** If the person says "yes" you've got a deal. If the person says "no," ask, "Would you help me think of someone who can help me?" You might say, "Would you help me find some other way to get what I need?"

You will more than likely get a positive response. If not, this person is not your friend. Find someone else who knows how to be a friend.

▷ **Step 10:** Use this same approach in many areas of your life to make living a lot easier.

This approach is especially helpful for people who are dealing with ADD. Ask someone who is farther along than you to give you a helping hand. This is what a mentor can do.

Later you will have the opportunity to pass what you have learned on down the line to the newcomers who are just beginning to learn what do about their ADD.

CUTTING A DEAL

With attention deficit disorder (or anything else for that matter), it is very useful to learn to cut deals and make trades so that you can take advantage of your assets and get help with your liabilities.

Make a list of everyday-living skills that you have, such as mechanical ability, bookkeeping, cooking, or creative talent.

I can

_____   _____

_____   _____

_____   _____

_____   _____

List areas in which you need help.

_____   _____

_____   _____

_____   _____

Who do you know who has talent in an area in which you need help?

_____

_____

_____

Ask those people if they would be willing to make a trade with you. Say, "I need help with my bookkeeping." Make an offer to trade one of your skills in return. Say, "I could cook dinner for your family one evening a month in exchange. Would you be interested?"

If you are turned down, ask whether it is because the person doesn't want to do the job or doesn't need what you offered. Then ask if there is something that person does need. Ask for a suggestion. Say, "Is there something you need that I might be able to supply?" Don't forget to offer money if you have it to trade.

Sometimes trading responsibility for an undesired job is necessary. For example:

Say, "Since neither one of us wants to cut the grass, how would you feel if I did it one week and you did it the next?" Or you both might decide that neither of you wants to cut the grass and you will each work a few extra hours of overtime so that you can pay someone to do it.

Be sure that no one loses in any of these negotiations. They *must* be done with no coercion or power plays. And remember, a deal is only as good as the honesty of the people making it.

► Consensus, Not Compromise

When two people have differences, they must figure out some way to resolve those differences. Otherwise the relationship can be threatened when

- ▷ tempers rise
- ▷ stress takes over
- ▷ verbal battles occur
- ▷ attempts are made to determine who is right and who is wrong
- ▷ one person pressures the other into a one-sided solution

Two problem-solving methods are common. One uses compromise; the other tries to reach a consensus.

COMPROMISE

Typically people think about compromising when they run into difficulty as they attempt to solve a problem. With compromise, however, no one get what he wants. Both people lose out. For example, let's suppose you want Chinese food while your spouse wants Mexican food. If you compromise so that you resolve the impasse by getting Italian food, which neither of you really wants, neither of you gets what you want. Each of you shares a loss.

CONSENSUS

With consensus, both people agree to find a solution that each truly wants—at no loss to either. Each person agrees to continue to seek a solution until *both* are pleased.

Important factors

- ▷ No sense of loss
- ▷ No power plays
- ▷ No giving in

125

The results of consensus
  ▷ A sense of fairness
  ▷ An opportunity to work in each other's best interest
  ▷ A sense of achievement for a shared solution

If you would like to get these results, proceed.

▷ **Step 1:** Think of a situation in which you and another person have a difference to resolve.

▷ **Step 2:** Write down as many solutions as you can think of. If possible, do this with the person with whom you have the difference.

_____

_____

_____

_____

If you cannot come up with something that is mutually satisfying to both of you, you may need to consider an alternative such as picking up food at both a Mexican and a Chinese restaurant and then taking it to the park.

▷ **Step 3:** If you are not able to agree, ask some friends to join you. Their fresh approach may help. Add their suggestions.

_____

_____

_____

_____

If you still cannot come to a resolution, proceed.

▷ **Step 4:** You may need to agree to disagree. Then each of you may go your separate ways. In the case of the food example, you may simply decide not to eat together that evening. A more sensitive issue is faced when one partner wants to have sex and the other does not. Then, simply feel the loving compassion that results from your having tried very hard to come to a solution together. Know that each of you did the best you could. Congratulations!

Communication is the backbone of relationships. Practice the skills listed here and know that, because of your extra sensitivity, you can have wonderful relationships.

▶ Interpersonal Intimacy

By definition, intimacy means having closeness in a relationship with another person. Three aspects of intimacy are important to define.

- ▷ The role you play in the relationship
- ▷ The type or form the intimacy takes
- ▷ The degree of intimacy or the limits surrounding it

ROLE

The role you play in relation to another is key in defining the relationship. Common roles include

- ▷ parent/child
- ▷ friend
- ▷ lover
- ▷ mentor
- ▷ teacher

TYPE

The close association can take many forms. It can mean

- ▷ deep understanding
- ▷ friendship
- ▷ brotherhood/sisterhood
- ▷ endearment
- ▷ love
- ▷ affection
- ▷ sexual intimacy

DEGREE

Limits help define the extent of involvement you want to have with the other person. This includes

- ▷ the amount of time you wish to spend together
- ▷ the intensity of relationship

It's up to you to define the three aspects. There is no right or wrong way to do this. *Your* definitions are dependent upon the role you wish to play in the relationship. The other person must do the same. Then, you compare your choices with each other to see how close the match is between you.

List here the people you feel close to, those you have affection for, and anyone with whom you are *in love.* After the person's name, note the type of connection: family, friend, lover, mentor, teacher, or other.

127

Name	Role	Type	Degree
_____	_____	_____	_____
_____	_____	_____	_____
_____	_____	_____	_____
_____	_____	_____	_____
_____	_____	_____	_____

Next, go back to the earlier list of types of intimacy. Choose the type that fits the relationship you have with each person you listed. List the type.

Finally, rate the intensity of the relationship. Ask yourself, "How much involvement do I want with this person; a lot, some, or a little bit?" Then mark the column headed "degree" with either, H (high), M (medium), or L (low).

Now you have a way of gaining clarity about your relationships. Instead of *them* happening *to you, you* can have some control in relation *to them.*

Expectations are one of the most difficult problems most people face in relationships. They involve what you want from another person and what you are willing to give to the other person. Similarly, what the other person wants or expects must be defined, as well as what that person can or will give to you.

When the form and limits of a relationship are clear, expectations are likely to be realistic. Therefore, you or your partner are less likely to get hurt or be disappointed.

EXPECTATIONS

Go back to the list on the previous page. Ask yourself,

"What do I want from the other person?"
"Does that person know what I want?"
"What does the person want from me?"
"Can I give it and do I want to give it?"

Be honest and clear with your answers to yourself. Share the results of this exercise with each person involved. Be sure to check your perceptions with the other person.

Say, "I believe you expect _____ from me. Is that accurate?"

Also ask, "Do you know I want _____ from you? Can you give it to me?"

▶ Responsibility and Intimacy

You may sometimes, or even always, feel inadequate, incomplete, or unacceptable. However, no one else can make up for the feeling of deficiency within you. Even when someone else wants to, it doesn't work. Only you can make the difference. However, **no one else can do the job as well as you can.**

By doing the job yourself, you take responsibility for yourself. If that feels impossible because of feelings of inadequacy and the like, know that you can learn. To learn how, continue.

SELF-RESPONSIBILITY

Being self-responsible has two aspects to it.

▷ In relation to your perception of yourself
▷ In relation to your perception of others

In relation to your perception of yourself, ask the following:

Have I often felt inadequate?

_____ yes _____ no

Where did I feel inadequate?

_____ in relationships _____ in school _____ at work

Do I feel incomplete without someone else around?

_____ yes _____ no

Do I wonder what others see in me?

_____ yes _____ no

Have I often felt rejected or unacceptable and felt it was my fault?

_____ yes _____ no

"Yes" responses to these questions indicate that you probably formed a negative picture of yourself. It is time to change that.

▷ **Step 1:** Know that everyone has strengths and weaknesses.
▷ **Step 2:** Realize that you know about your weaknesses but do not know about other's weaknesses.

▷ **Step 3:** Know that you are aware of other's strengths but do not know about your own.

▷ **Step 4:** Make a list of your strengths. Get someone to help you make a long list.

_____	_____
_____	_____
_____	_____
_____	_____
_____	_____

▷ **Step 5:** Be willing to acknowledge your strengths. Say, "I am _____." (list your strengths)

▷ **Step 6:** Then affirm your willingness to *learn* to be self-responsible. Say, "I am willing to be responsible for myself."

▷ **Step 7:** Affirm your ability to learn. Say, "I can learn to be responsible."

▷ **Step 8:** If you feel scared that you won't be able to learn or that you will fail, say, "I remember times when I failed to do what I wanted to do. I now know that I have grown and can succeed. I release my fears."

▷ **Step 9:** Say, "I have or can get help to do this learning while still staying responsible for myself."

Before going further with your learning to be self-responsible, look at the roles that others play in relation to you.

In relation to your perception of others, ask the following:

Do you feel others know what is better for you than you know for yourself?

_____ yes   _____ no

Are you told by others that they know what is best for you?

_____ yes   _____ no

Do you let others take care of you?

_____ yes   _____ no

Do you let others do things for you that you could actually do for yourself?

_____ yes   _____ no

Do you believe that someone else's way is better than your way?

_____ yes _____ no

"Yes" responses indicate that you are putting responsibility for yourself in another person or that you've allowed another person to take responsibility for you.

Anytime you give another person power over you, you make them responsible for you or a part of your life. This includes times when you elevate their way of doing things above your way.

Others cannot do the job *for* you but they can do it *with* you. You do not need to work in isolation. You just need to mentally take responsibility for yourself and your actions and *ask* others to help you. They also need to have the right of refusal. No one is obligated to help you. To change your perception of others' role in your life, proceed.

▷ **Step 1:** Repeat, "No one has responsibility for me or my life."
▷ **Step 2:** List the people who are taking responsibility for parts of your life. This could include waking you up in the morning, doing your checkbook, paying your bills, bailing you out of trouble (financial, legal, or other), or serving as entertainment director for your time off.

Name   Responsibility

_____   _____

_____   _____

_____   _____

▷ **Step 3:** Go back over the list and determine whether you and the other person ever made an agreement for the other person to take that responsibility.
▷ **Step 4:** Ask yourself whether you have outgrown the agreement. Are you now capable or willing to do more than you did before for yourself?
▷ **Step 5:** Return to the person and reassess your needs and the deal you made earlier. Take all the responsibility you are able to at this time.
▷ **Step 6:** Thank the person for the help given thus far.
▷ **Step 7:** Thank yourself for being honest now. Give yourself a pat on the back.
▷ **Step 8:** If the person continues to take responsibility for your business, resist. Walk away if you must. Be kind but firm, saying, "I'll handle it."

Now you can continue to grow, which is what happens when you take as much responsibility as you are capable of taking.

More power to you!

Continue to talk to yourself about being responsible. Be willing to affirm that you are no longer a kid (no matter what your age).

Say,

"I am no longer a kid."

"I am an adult."

"I can count on myself to follow through."

"I am in charge of myself."

"I'm pretty terrific."

▶ Limits

Limits define and express the extent of our responsibility and power. They

- ▷ show others and ourselves what we are willing to do or accept.
- ▷ act as a protection.
- ▷ make boundaries for us to follow so we know what someone else wants or needs.

Limits need to be

- ▷ clearly stated.
- ▷ consistently applied.
- ▷ fairly equal in relation to the other person. That is, the limits you place on another need to be close to the limits placed upon you by that other person. Otherwise, the relationship is unbalanced.
- ▷ respected even if you don't agree with them.

If someone has placed limits on you, ask the following questions:

Do I feel trapped by another's limits?

_____ yes   _____ no

Am I willing to go along with the limits imposed by another person?

_____ yes   _____ no

Do I seem to be unable to live up to the limits another imposes?

_____ yes   _____ no

Do I try and fail?

_____ yes   _____ no

Do I intend to comply but find I'm unable to do the job?

_____ yes   _____ no

OTHERS' LIMITS ON YOU

Having limits placed on you by another person puts you in the position of deciding whether you *want* to accept those limits or not. To make that decision, take the following steps.

▷ **Step 1:** Think about the cost to you of the limits. For example, your wife handles the family's finances including seeing that you stick to the budget. So she set a limit of how much you can spend. One cost of the budget limit might be that you feel like a child. Another cost could be that she feels irritability because she really doesn't want to be responsible for keeping you on the budget.

▷ **Step 2:** Ask yourself what you gain by complying with the limits. To find the answer you might ask yourself, "Would I lose something if I chose not to accept the limits?" You might feel as if you would lose control of your finances without your wife helping. That means you gain a sense of security about your money from letting your wife take responsibility for keeping you on the budget.

▷ **Step 3:** Assess in your mind whether that is too high a price for you to pay for your sense of security. Maybe it is; maybe it's not.

▷ **Step 4:** If the price is too high, look for an alternative way to gain a feeling of security that doesn't cost as much emotionally. One example might be for you to take over the responsibility for the management of your money. You might separate the money from your pay check into envelopes that cover different kinds of expenses: food, entertainment, and so forth. Then make the commitment *never* to shift money from one envelope to another. Or you might give yourself permission to hire a bookkeeper who will keep you on track.

▷ **Step 5:** Talk the changes over with the other person after you have a plan to present. That way you stay in charge of you, which is important because no one knows as well as you do what is best for you. And, *you deserve to be in charge of your life!*

SETTING LIMITS ON OTHERS

Placing limits on another person is an important skill to gain. It aids others in knowing what you expect and what you would like in a relationship. Limits also let you protect yourself, which is very important in becoming a responsible person.

In order to set constructive limits, follow these steps:

▷ **Step 1:** Decide what you *want* to do or what you are *willing* to do. Either figure it out in your own mind or talk with someone who is not involved in your situation. Suppose you are willing to be on the board of directors at your church *but* are not willing to head up a committee that will take a lot of extra time.

▷ **Step 2:** Initiate a discussion about what you desire. Do not wait until others make assumptions about what you will or won't do. First say what you are willing to do. "I am willing to be on the board of directors."

▷ **Step 3:** Immediately speak of the limitations on what you've already said. "I will not be able, however, to chair a committee."

▷ **Step 4:** Then, offer the opportunity for the other person to respond to your limit. "I understand that you might need to find someone who can do both." Just be up front about your needs and limitations. Honesty is the best policy.

Do not be afraid that people will fail to like you because you set limits. Sometimes people will not like *what* you do but that doesn't mean they don't like you. Make it okay for them to make this distinction.

▷ **Step 1:** Say, "I'm sorry to let you down. I can imagine that you might feel irritated or disappointed with me, but I did not intend to cause you difficulty. This is something I need to do for myself."

▷ **Step 2:** You might want to help the person find another solution to the problem. "Let me think about who might be free to give you a helping hand on the board. I'll put some thought into it and give you a call by Friday."

▷ **Step 3:** Finally, thank the person for his understanding.

If someone expresses anger when you set a limit, *recognize* their feelings but do not give way to the feelings. Say, "I see that you are angry, but I still must do what I feel is the best for me." Or you might say, "If you need to be angry with my decision, I understand, but I must do what I need to do for myself. It is not my intent to cause you trouble."

You may need to set limits on the anger if the person cannot let go of it. For example, "I realize you are angry. I've heard you but I cannot help you further. I'm leaving until you feel better." This direct approach is for use when someone goes on and on and on. There is no constructive reason to continue to allow yourself to listen to the anger or to let the person continue to spew the anger out.

▶ Sexual Intimacy

Of all the forms of intimacy, sexual closeness between two people can be the most difficult to handle in a healthy, constructive way. Sexual expression as the outgrowth of a close, enjoyable connection between two people can be misunderstood, misapplied, or hurtful.

Answer the following questions to determine the patterns of your personal intimacy.

Does intimacy automatically mean sexual intimacy to you?

_____ yes _____ no

Do sex and affection seem the same to you?

_____ yes _____ no

Does the expression of affection always lead to sex?

_____ yes _____ no

Does sex serve other purposes than to express love?

_____ yes _____ no

Do you want sex to relieve tension?

_____ yes _____ no

At times do you crave sex compulsively?

_____ yes _____ no

Are you never satisfied no matter how much or what kind of sex you have?

_____ yes _____ no

135

Is it hard for you to find different ways to enjoy sex with a partner you care a lot about?

_____ yes _____ no

Do you sometimes satisfy your sexual desires at the expense of another person?

_____ yes _____ no

Do you feel cheated when your sexual partner is unavailable to satisfy your sexual desires?

_____ yes _____ no

The more "yes" responses you have, the more likely you are to be struggling with a use of sex that is likely to lead you and your partner to frustration. Emotionally healthy sex

- ▷ is fulfilling for both partners.
- ▷ is the natural outgrowth of a loving, caring, committed relationship.
- ▷ is an extension of an expression of affection for another to whom you are drawn sexually.
- ▷ communicates respect for another.
- ▷ honors the needs and desires of both partners.
- ▷ is never hurtful or disrespectful.
- ▷ is fun and rewarding much of the time.

COMMON MISUNDERSTANDINGS ABOUT SEX

Myth: Affection leads to sex automatically.
Correction: Sometimes expressions of affection lead to sex. Sometimes affection is an end in itself.

To change your misconception do the following:

▷ **Step 1:** Ask your partner what he or she feels about the relationship between sex and affection.

Write the response here_____

_____

_____

_____

_____

_____

▷ **Step 2:** Ask yourself where you first learned your ideas about the relationship between sex and affection.

Write your response here _____

_____

_____

_____

_____

_____

_____

▷ **Step 3:** Begin to experiment with little signs of affection so you can separate the two behaviors. Ask your partner what he or she likes. Remember, affection is often an expression of nurturing, support, and caring. A pat on the shoulder or a hug may do a world of good for your partner. Try it.

▷ **Step 4:** Remind yourself that this show of affection does not have to do with sex or sexuality. Tell yourself, "That's different."

▷ **Step 5:** Another time, when you are feeling amorous, let your partner know clearly. Tell him or her that romance is on your mind. That way you will be clear about the end goal of the affection you show under these circumstances.

MISAPPLICATION: TO FEED AN ADDICTION

Sex used for purposes other than the mutual expression of love can be an addiction. Such addictions often form as the result of the premature introduction of sex in inappropriate situations. Or the partner may have crossed lines of acceptable behavior based on the primary role being played by the person. An example would be a teacher who seduced a young student or a child who was sexually abused by an older child.

Correction: Sex is a physical and emotional expression of love and caring between two consenting adults who choose to be with each other in this manner.

To change:

▷ **Step 1:** You may want to seek assistance from a counselor with this part of your development. Sometimes a good, nonjudgmental friend can help you, too. Also, there are support groups in many communities for people who have sexual addiction problems.

▷ **Step 2:** Think about what your attitudes about sex are.

Write here _____

_____

_____

_____

▷ **Step 3:** From whom did you learn them?

Write here _____

_____

_____

_____

▷ **Step 4:** What attitudes would you like to have now?

Write here _____

_____

_____

_____

▷ **Step 5:** What are the needs of the part of you who experienced the inappropriate introduction to sex?

Write here _____

_____

_____

_____

This may be the time to make use of a counselor who can help you make the situation feel right. You deserve to be healed and protected and to be free to enjoy yourself fully in relationships.

▷ **Step 6:** If you are ready, forgive all involved in the earlier experience. If that does not feel comfortable for you, do not push yourself. But do get help. You deserve it.

MISAPPLICATION: FOR THE WRONG REASONS

Correction: Using sex to cover fears, anxieties, low self esteem, or any other emotional inadequacies is giving sex a job that it was never intended to do. Learn to manage the inadequacies directly and relieve sex of that burden. Then it can be enjoyed for what it is.

To change:

▷ **Step 1:** Ask yourself how you want to use your sexuality.

Write here _____

_____

_____

_____

▷ **Step 2:** List the various ways you become sexually aroused such as looking at pictures, making use of prostitutes, having affairs, exposing yourself, and so on.

Write here _____

_____

_____

_____

_____

▷ **Step 3:** How does each of these ways make you feel?

Write here _____

_____

_____

_____

_____

▷ **Step 4:** Look for other ways to get the feelings you desire rather than through sexuality. You may need a counselor or support group to help you with this. List them below.

Write here _____

_____

_____

_____

MISAPPLICATION: TO DEMONSTRATE POWER OVER ANOTHER PERSON

Correction: Sex is given and received by permission only. It is never acceptable to force sex on another person. Psychological pressure as well as physical force are not acceptable.

To change:

▷ **Step 1:** Ask yourself, "Who forced you to do things when you were young?"

Write here _____

_____

_____

▷ **Step 2:** Remember, that was then. Forcing someone now does not fix the situation then. It will probably take a counselor to help you deal with the past.

▷ **Step 3:** Make a commitment to keep the past and the present separate. Say, "I commit to let the past be the past, to get help with it, and to live the present with a clear mind."

▷ **Step 4:** Get a buddy whom you commit to contact when you begin to feel angry or tense in the present time. Do not translate those feelings into action.

I choose _____

MISAPPLICATION: TO RELIEVE TENSION

Correction: Use sex for the right reasons. Sex is for the mutual expression of two people's feelings for each other. Stress can be dealt with in many ways other than by using sex.

To change:

▷ **Step 1:** Think about the last time you used sex to relieve tension.

▷ **Step 2:** Let yourself feel what it felt like to be stressed. Become clear about how you experience stress. Ask yourself the following:

How do I feel the tension physically?_____

_____

_____

In what part of my body do I feel it? _____

_____

_____

Emotionally, how do I experience stress?_____

_____

_____

What happens to my thinking when I am under stress? _____

_____

_____

▷ **Step 3:** As you become aware of stress, physically, emotionally, or cognitively, stop what you are doing and *decide* what you want to do to alleviate the stress. Go to the section on stress for suggestions.

▷ **Step 4:** Take care of the stress right away.

▷ **Step 5:** Build your awareness of what works for you as a tension reliever.

▷ **Step 6:** Begin to build regular tension reduction time into your daily living. This way it won't build up. Rather, you will head off the accumulation of tension.

▷ **Step 7:** Once you have ways to deal with stress in your life, you can turn your attention to enjoying sex for the communication with another person that it brings you.

► Healthy Sexual Intimacy and ADD

Mutually expressive sexuality can bring joy, pleasure, and fun into a relationship. Part play, part sweetness, part excitement, and part tenderness, sexual communication between two people is one aspect of a healthy union. To be certain that sexual intimacy brings these pleasures to you, consider the following factors:

▷ timing
▷ telling
▷ touch
▷ thank you

Understanding the role that each of these factors plays in your sexual experience is the first step. Learning how to be skillful in the implementation of each is the second. The rewards are many and worth spending a bit of time becoming proficient.

TIMING

People with ADD often have difficulty with time management, getting to places on time, or being distracted. Timing, however, is different. Knowing how and when to approach a person is important. Knowing how much is enough or too much is imperative. Knowing when to stop, back off, or continue with sexual behavior is a skill you can acquire.

Your ADD Is an Asset: Sensitivity to other people's feelings and needs is a part of ADD.

Ask yourself the following:

Do you know when you or your special other has had enough of a certain touch or move?

_____ yes   _____ no

Can you tell whether your timing and level of desire match your partner's so that you reach satisfaction together or at nearly the same time?

_____ yes   _____ no

To make sure you are getting your timing down do the following:

▷ **Step 1:** Pay attention for a little while to the needs, desires, and timing of your partner. Also do the same for yourself.
▷ **Step 2:** Become aware of your moods and the moods of your partner.
▷ **Step 3:** Do not do anything sexually that begins to bore you or that makes you uncomfortable or restless.
▷ **Step 4:** When you've had enough, say so. "I've had all I want for now. I love you, but I'm not comfortable with any more."
▷ **Step 5:** Be sure to accommodate your partner in the same way.

Many people with attention deficit disorder do not like prolonged periods of foreplay or sexual activity. That does not mean they are unloving. Nor does it mean they don't love their partners. Their timing is simply different from that of someone who likes to spend a lot of time making love.

TELLING

It is imperative to communicate with your sexual partner about what you do and don't like. In all likelihood you and your partner are different with regard to what you each like and don't like.

▷ **Step 1:** Make a list of what makes you feel good sexually.

Write here _____

_____

_____

_____

▷ **Step 2:** Ask your sexual partner to do the same. (Cover up your list so your partner can't see what you wrote.)

Write here _____

_____

_____

_____

_____

▷ **Step 3:** Now trade lists and share what you wrote.

▷ **Step 4:** Interview each other about what feels the very best, what you would like occasionally, and what you like a lot but for short periods of time.

▷ **Step 5:** Now each of you make a list of what bothers you or what you do not like.

▷ **Step 6:** Similarly, share these lists and interview each other.

▷ **Step 7:** Agree to practice with each other soon to experience firsthand what you've just shared.

▷ **Step 8:** During the sexual encounter, be sure to communicate your feelings, your preferences, and your needs.

▷ **Step 9:** Be cautious that you do not take each other for granted. Continue to talk indefinitely, letting each other know how pleased you are to be able to please one another.

▷ **Step 10:** Periodically explore new and different ways of making love. Enjoy yourselves.

TOUCH

People who have ADD generally have finely tuned sensory systems. It would not be surprising if your sense of touch is very keen. You can use that to advantage. It can also make you feel awful. To achieve positive results, follow these steps.

▷ **Step 1:** Become aware of how you like to be touched. Do you want to be patted, stroked, tickled? How long do you like the touching to continue?

▷ **Step 2:** Communicate your preferences to your partner.

▷ **Step 3:** Remember that nothing is good or bad when it comes to sexual expression. As long as you have permission from the other person to be sexually active and neither of you acts in a hurtful way, you can have free reign to enjoy yourselves.

▷ **Step 4:** If you do not like prolonged touching, don't forget that your partner may. Offer to please your partner even if you no longer want to be made love to.

143

▷ **Step 5:** Be kind to one another. Do not insist on always having your way. Learn to be generous to each other but honest, so that you don't become resentful or angry.

Your sexual activity can be one of the most pleasant aspects of your life. Share generously, take responsibility for yourself, and be open and receptive to the needs of your partner. Remember, ADD can be an asset as well as a liability. Just remember to communicate about it. May the pleasure be yours.

Chapter 5
Living Up to Your Potential

Potential! A word that may cause chills to run though your body. Yet the only reason anxiety and discomfort surround the word is the fear of not being able to live up to potential. And no one suffers more from that loss of potential than the person with ADD.

The good news is that you now know enough to be able to reach your potential. Key factors to realize.

▷ Potential does not disappear if it is unreached.
▷ Your body, mind, and spirit are forever searching for ways to exercise it.
▷ At any time you can manifest its expression.
▷ Knowing what ADD is about allows you to overcome the blocks that previously deterred you from being all you could be.

You must know that

▷ if you can dream it, you can do it.
▷ what you admire in others you already have in yourself.

If you would like to learn how to reach your potential, proceed.

Ask yourself the following:

Am I willing to give myself permission to be someone who has her/his ADD under control?

_____ yes   _____ no

Am I ready to invite my identity to change now that I know why I was the way I was before I discovered I have ADD?

_____ yes   _____ no

Am I ready to recognize my potential?

_____ yes   _____ no

145

Dare I hope that I can reach my potential?

_____ yes   _____ no

Answering "yes" to these questions means you are ready to make a change. It's up to you! If you want to update your identity, proceed.

▷ **Step 1:** Say "goodbye" to the pre-diagnosis ADD identity. Visualize yourself during that time and realize you did the best you could.
▷ **Step 2:** Grieve if you feel like it.
▷ **Step 3:** Release the old beliefs that held you down.
▷ **Step 4:** Be prepared to live between the old and the new identities for a time. It is necessary to release the old image, habits, and beliefs before the new ones can move into place.
▷ **Step 5:** While you are waiting, be aware of what you like and dislike, want and don't want, desire and hope for.
▷ **Step 6:** Keep alert to the newly emerging you and make note of your newly forming identity.

Realize there are many stages to discovering your identity now that you have your ADD under control. It can be an exciting adventure. If you would like to find out more, go to the next section.

▶ What Am I Like? Before and After

There are many beliefs, attitudes, and perceptions that you have had about yourself that may begin to change. You can learn a lot about yourself by contrasting your old identity with your new one.

To begin this process, answer the following questions:

How did you see yourself physically (before you had your ADD under control)? _____

_____

_____

How do you see yourself physically (now that you have your ADD under control)? _____

_____

_____

How did you see yourself emotionally? _____

_____

_____

How do you see yourself emotionally? _____

_____

_____

How did you see yourself intellectually? _____

_____

_____

How do you see yourself intellectually? _____

_____

_____

How did you see yourself spiritually? _____

_____

_____

How do you see yourself spiritually? _____

_____

_____

What are your greatest strengths? _____

_____

_____

What are your greatest vulnerabilities? _____

_____

_____

What has changed most about you? _____

_____

_____

How do you like change? _____

_____

_____

How do you feel about stability? _____

_____

_____

Contrasting how you were before your ADD was under control with how you are now may have proved insightful to you. Whenever you are considering your identity, be sure to check your feelings. Notice whether or not you felt happy, light, and excited about the way in which you see yourself. Note the changes and proceed to discover more about you now.

▶ Who Am I?

To help you clarify your new identity, consider what you like and dislike. The following list of your favorites and least favorites may help you to discover more about yourself. Answer them thoughtfully rather than automatically. Remember, as your identity shifts, so may your interests. Be sure your responses are up to date. You may even want to do some experimenting to figure out what you now like.

Feel free to leave any space blank or substitute any topic that has appeal for you. Pay attention to how you feel as you do this. Note how intense your feelings are.

Item	Favorite	Least Favorite
Food		
Meal time		
Flower		
Color		
Animal		
Mode of transportation		
Fantasy mode of transportation		
Sport (participant)		
Sport (to observe)		
Type of social activity		
Type of social setting (clubs, out-of-doors, etc.)		
Type of friend		

Item	Favorite	Least Favorite
Way to spend money		
Movie/TV show/Play		
Actor/Actress		
Book/Written material		
Music		
Electronic Game		
Art/craft		
Hobby		
Silly thing to do		
Vacation spot		
Place to live		
Kind of home		
Season		
Time of day		
Work setting		
Place to work (city, home, etc.)		
Style of clothing		

Add any more that you want that will give you an idea of what you like these days.

As you filled in your favorites and least favorites, what did you feel? Go back over the list.

1. With a red pencil, check the items that stand out as special favorites, the ones you absolutely want in your life. Commit to include them in your life. Even though you may not immediately be able to implement some of them, you can hold the image of your desire in your mind to continue to work toward.

2. Draw a line through the responses that you dislike a lot and commit to eliminate them from your life. There is no need for you to waste your time on anything that does not fit you. You have enough to do to implement your new identity. Enjoy the task.

Now that you've gotten a new sense about some of the aspects of your likes and dislikes, look at yourself in some other ways. Answer the following questions:

149

On a daily basis what would you like to do more of?_____

_____

In what setting do you feel most effective?_____

_____

_____

What do you need to be more effective? _____

_____

_____

What can you not keep from doing? _____

_____

_____

▶ Your Job and Your Potential

As more of your identity unfolds, as your confidence builds, and as you begin to truly believe you can measure up to your potential, you can allow yourself to expand your sense of self into all the aspects of your life. And a major part of your life is the workplace. If you would like to take a closer look at your identity in relation to your work, continue.

Several factors contribute to selecting a work environment that fits you.

- ▷ self employment vs. working for someone
- ▷ size of business or company
- ▷ setting of job (city/small town/country)
- ▷ type of supervisor or boss preferred
- ▷ intensity of job environment

The task of investigating the type and style of work environment that fits you demands that you know yourself. Again it is important to monitor your feelings as you respond to the options because your feelings will tell you what fits you. If you feel relaxed, happy, even excited, you will know you are on the right track for you. If you feel tense, irritable, or sad, you will know you are on the wrong one.

Ask yourself the following:

Would I like to work for myself?

_____ yes   _____ no

Would I prefer to work for someone?

_____ yes _____ no

Do I like the idea of being a part of a big company?

_____ yes _____ no

Would I like to work for a corporation?

_____ yes _____ no

Would I like to work in a small company?

_____ yes _____ no

Do I prefer the idea of working in the city?

_____ yes _____ no

Would I rather be in a small town?

_____ yes _____ no

Would I like to be in the country?

_____ yes _____ no

Do I prefer a boss who is laid back?

_____ yes _____ no

Would I like a boss who motivates me?

_____ yes _____ no

Do I need someone who is very structured and sticks to the letter of the law?

_____ yes _____ no

Would I like to work with a partner?

_____ yes _____ no

151

What kind of partner would I like in terms of personality?

_____

_____

What kind of partner would I like in terms of skill? _____

_____

_____

Would I prefer a relaxed work environment?

_____ yes _____ no

Would I rather have a formal work environment?

_____ yes _____ no

Would I rather work inside?

_____ yes _____ no

Would I prefer to be out-of-doors?

_____ yes _____ no

Do I need and want variety on the job?

_____ yes _____ no

Would I prefer to do the same things daily?

_____ yes _____ no

These questions will give you a good idea of the type of work setting you prefer. No one setting is better or worse. They are only different. In order to increase the odds that you will be working in a manner and style that fits you, follow these steps.

▷ **Step 1:** Make a list of the characteristics that you discovered you would like to have in a job.

_____   _____

_____   _____

_____   _____

_____   _____

▷ **Step 2:** Write a description of the work setting that you
would prefer.

▷ **Step 3:** Be sure that you don't jump to conclusions about
why you cannot have what you want. During this
stage all you have to do is expand your awareness of
what you prefer. Do not go further at this time.

By now, you have an initial idea of what you like and dislike and the settings in which you are likely to function best.

How you make your living and express yourself are crucial to how you feel about yourself. To expand your awareness
into this area of your life, continue.

What do you need from a job to feel successful? _____

_____

_____

_____

What would you need from a job to feel wonderful? _____

_____

_____

_____

What is your "heart" job? (A heart job is one that makes your
heart sing. It's one that so fits who and what you are that you
want to get up on Monday morning to do it, or one that you
would do whether you were paid or not.)

_____

_____

_____

_____

You may have trouble answering the last question if it is
premature, that is, you may not be ready to answer it yet.
That's okay. Go on ahead to answer the following questions.
Then come back to it.

► Dream Time

Your ability to dream is a mighty tool to use in finding out
about yourself. It's time to "go for broke." Proceed to expand
your self-awareness.

What is your secret dream? _____

_____

_____

_____

_____

_____

_____

If you had a magic wand so that you could make anything happen—
you could have all the money you needed and wanted, instant
education and skills, the ability to create whatever you needed or
wanted—what would you want to do with your time?

_____

_____

_____

_____

_____

_____

If you won the lottery or sweepstakes, what would you choose to do
with your time?

_____

_____

_____

_____

_____

Now, consider your heart job. Return to page 153 and complete the
question.

By dreaming, you can gain a fuller idea of who you are so
that by now you probably have a fairly good idea of who you
are or could be in the workplace.

If you are interested in going one step further, consider
that you can live your life any way that you want. You *can* live
any way you want. To explore further, consider the following
questions.

What would you love to do with your life? _____

_____

_____

_____

_____

_____

If you could be a full-time volunteer, how would you spend your time?

_____

_____

_____

_____

_____

What five people do you most admire and why? (They can be alive or dead, real or fantasy, known to you or strangers.)

1. _____

_____

2. _____

_____

3. _____

_____

4. _____

_____

5. _____

_____

What kind of person would you like to be? _____

_____

_____

_____

_____

_____

What would you like to contribute to humanity through your life? (Any answer is okay, including nothing.)

_____

_____

_____

_____

How would you like to be remembered? _____

_____

_____

_____

What would you like inscribed on your tombstone? _____

_____

_____

▶ Your ADD and Your Potential

Having ADD can be both an asset and a liability. Many favorable characteristics that can help you achieve your dreams and goals in life can be directly traced to the fact that ADD is a part of your life. Following is a list of ADD characteristics that are often considered favorable. How many do you have?

_____ Sensitive

_____ Expressive

_____ Empathetic in relation to others (feel what they feel)

_____ Feel deeply

_____ Creative (including problem solving, the way you look at things, as well as how you live day by day)

_____ Inventive

_____ See things from a unique perspective

_____ Perceptually aware, observant

_____ Spontaneous

_____ Humorous

_____ Fun

_____ Energetic

_____ Open, not secretive

_____ Eager for acceptance and willing to work for it

_____ Responsive to positive reinforcement

_____ Do not harbor resentment

_____ More likely to do what you want than what you should

_____ Operate more from your heart than your head

_____ Read people well

_____ Look past surface appearances to the core of people, situations, and issues

_____ Down to earth

_____ Good networker

_____ Sees unique relationships between people and things

_____ Can take an interdisciplinary approach to things

_____ Not likely to get in a rut

_____ Original

_____ Loyal

_____ Intense when interested in something

_____ Quick, if you like what you are doing

After considering these traits, go back to your dreams and see which traits fit which dreams. You will find that you have a head start. More power to you.

Now, consider how your ADD can get in the way of developing your dreams. In the following, select a dream with which you would like to work.

The dream that I choose is_____

_____

_____

Now, make note of the ADD traits that you are concerned will get in the way.

_____   _____

_____   _____

_____   _____

Next, go to the sections of the workbook that deal with these traits and work at overcoming their negative effects on your life.

You can do it! And realize that, as you do, your dreams become your potential.

▶ Training to Your Potential

Knowing better who you are and what you want and don't want to do, you are now in a position to set priorities. Remember, you can have it all—maybe just not at once.

▷ **Step 1:** Answer the following questions.

Do I want/need to establish an income base that will support me and any other people for whom I choose to be responsible?

_____ yes _____ no

Do I want to strive for my heart job immediately?

_____ yes _____ no

Do I want to commit to pursue my heart job at the same time that I develop an immediate income base?

_____ yes _____ no

One of the most important parts of answering these questions is to pay attention to how you feel as you answer them. You may notice where you feel strained. That means you are giving an answer that you think you should give but it does not really fit you. When you feel happy or excited answering a question, you will know you are doing something that is in your best interest.

▷ **Step 2:** Select the choice with which you wish to begin.

I choose to begin by _____

_____

_____

This is your first goal.

▷ **Step 3:** Use what you learned in order to break down long-range projects on page 101. List the components involved in developing this project. Be sure to include the need to gather more information or experience in order to wisely make a long-range plan.

▷ **Step 4:** Order the components in a step-by-step plan to reach your goal.

▷ **Step 5:** Check your plan with a trusted friend, colleague, mentor, or counselor who will support you and help you achieve an orderly plan that you can successfully complete in order to reach your goal.

▷ **Step 6:** Establish a time frame. To do this, consider how much time you have available to work each day or week on your plan. It doesn't matter how much you choose. Rather, it's important to want to spend the amount of time you choose so you will do it. (Hint: Do not exceed the amount of time you list here by very much without revising your operating plan. Otherwise, you are letting the project run you rather than you being in charge of it. You also run the risk of burning out.)

▶ Keeping on Track

For you to reach your potential, it is critical that you keep on track. That does not mean that you have to work rigidly at the same time daily, or that if you fall off the track all is lost.

In order to keep on track, follow these steps.

▷ **Step 1:** Have a regular time to assess the headway you are making in relation to your goal. You may want to go over it with your mentor or other helper.

Do not assess your progress too frequently or you may be unable to accomplish enough to make you feel good. On the other hand, do not allow too much time to go by so that you get so far off track that it feels difficult to get back on.

Use the following list to help you assess your progress. Place a check by each item completed.

_____ I've gathered the components of my project together.

_____ I've gathered the following information about those components.

_____

_____

_____

_____

_____

_____

159

I've stayed on track with the following steps of my project.

_____ Step_____

_____ Step_____

_____ Step_____

_____ Step_____

_____ Step_____

My timing is okay _____ ahead _____ behind _____

Adjust your timing accordingly. You may wish to reassess the amount of time you thought you had available to do the project. Remember it is more important to stay in line with your timing than to reach the goal more quickly or slowly than you had planned.

If you've gotten off track, you need to reevaluate what you want to do, how you want to do it, and in what time. Ask what or who pulled you off track. And be sure to confer with someone else if that feels useful to you.

Ask yourself the following:

Do I still want to do this project?

_____ yes _____ no

Do I need to change the way I thought I would do the project?

_____ yes _____ no

Do I need to spend more time on the project?

_____ yes _____ no

Do I need to spend less time on the project?

_____ yes _____ no

Have I allowed someone to distract me from the project?

_____ yes _____ no

Have I allowed something to distract me from it?

_____ yes _____ no

Why have I allowed this to happen? _____

_____

_____

Am I afraid to say "no" to people?

_____ yes   _____ no

Do I doubt the decisions and steps I'm taking?

_____ yes   _____ no

Do I need to talk with someone I trust to feel better about my plan?

_____ yes   _____ no

Am I allowing someone to erode my confidence in the project or my ability to pull it off? (Some people cannot stand to see others succeed. This is especially true if you have come from an environment where you were seen as "the one who has the problem." In the process of changing your identity, you must realize that others have to change their perceptions of you.

▷ **Step 2:** Once you've assessed your progress, it's time to bolster yourself and assure your forward movement. To counteract some of the negative influences you may have encountered, consider the following ways to take control of yourself and the project.

Ask for what you want.
Ask for what you want, clearly, without a lot of explanation and apology. Give enough information for the person to know what you want.

Make direct requests.
Say, "I want access to your files. Will you give it to me?" Limit yourself to a short explanation of two or three sentences. If the answer is "no," say, "Thank you for considering my request."

Learn to say "no."
Do not hedge or beat around the bush. Just say "no."

You also need to take control of your situation when other people are involved. Consider using the following "power lines" when you are dealing with the pressure from and in relation to others. Use them as affirmations. Put them on your refrigerator or the dashboard of your car.

You Have the Right to Put Yourself First.
You've Got to Ask for What You Want.
Stay in Control with Controlling People.
Be Protective: There Really Are Bad Guys Out There.
Watch Your Boundaries.
"No" Is the Most Powerful Word You'll Ever Use.
You Have a Right to Your Own Choices.
Never Be Afraid to Ask.
Listen to Criticism, and Then Do What You Want.

Consider these power lines to empower yourself.

Take Responsibility for Solving Your Own Problems.
Life Is a Series of Problem-Solving Events.
You Can Always Count on Yourself.
Don't Do Things Because You're Afraid.
Take Control of Your Endings.
Take Care of Your Own Business First.
Stop, Look, and Listen When You're Blocked.
If You Can't Climb over the Mountain, Walk
    Around It.
You Do the Best You Can at Any Given Moment.
Respect Yourself.
Stick to It and You'll Do It.
Be Proud of Yourself.
Trust Yourself.
And finally,
There's No Such Thing as Failure.

Reward yourself every step of the way toward your goal and know that you cannot help but be who you are, and that is good. You cannot help but arrive at your goal as long as you keep after it. And, you cannot help but live up to your potential. You are a winner, you know.

Chapter 6
Continuing Your Education

► How to Survive

Continuing your education is a big step under any conditions. But for people with ADD, it can seem an enormous problem. You are likely to be discouraged by fear of failure, doubts about your intelligence, and concerns about your ability to meet the organizational demands of school. However, people with ADD can and do succeed in higher education. In fact, they frequently do better than when they were younger. You can, too.

But sometimes your mind may send you a different message. Listen to the self-talk that buzzes inside your head as you think about continuing your education. What do you hear? Typical messages sound something like this:

"I'll never be able to do well on tests."
"I'm the pretty one and my sister has the brains."
"It's no use. I always put things off until it's too late."
"I'm lazy."

If it is hard for you to believe that you can do better in school than you did when you were younger, write down the reasons why.

I feel discouraged because _____

and _____

and _____

Now, cross out those reasons and realize that you have changed and grown in many ways since the old school days. Remember:

▷ People with ADD can and do succeed in school.
▷ You can continue your education successfully.

163

> You can do better in school now than you did when you were younger because you

1. are more mature.
2. have discovered a special interest that holds your attention.
3. are able to apply practical, hands-on experience to your educational program.
4. can translate your special interest into a major, or can choose a school based on your special interest.
5. can learn to broker (get your needs met in) the education system.
6. can discover your special needs and learn to meet them.
7. are able to apply what you have learned from your practical, everyday living. (Remember, people with ADD learn by doing, so you have a wealth of knowledge gained by your experience.

While you are making your plans to return to school, you may find the exercises on the following pages helpful.

▶ Taking Stock of Your Maturity

Maturity is hard to define in everyday language. The dictionary defines it as "the state of being fully developed; perfected condition." Therefore, no one is ever completely mature, because no one is ever completely perfected. People with ADD often mature more slowly than others, but they get there just the same.

As you answer the questions on this page, keep in mind these points:

1) All around development (physical, intellectual, and emotional) tends to be slower in people who have ADD. Full maturity is reached but at a somewhat later age than your non-ADD counterparts.
2) A two- to five-year delay in reaching adulthood is not unusual. Ask yourself the following:

> Growing up, did you prefer to play with children younger than yourself?
> Did you sometimes feel that you just weren't ready to move on to the next grade or school level?
> Do you feel that too much is expected of you, or that you are given too much responsibility?

> ▷ Did you ever want to just take time off for a while before going on in school?
> ▷ Do you remember parents or teachers frequently telling you any of the following?

"Act your age," "Won't you ever grow up?" "You're acting like a baby," "Your little sister acts older than you," or "I ought to treat you like I do the babies." During childhood and adolescence, a few years' difference in development seems enormous. But later in life the same number of years seems immaterial. So do the following:

> ▷ Take your time. There is no reason to rush into more schooling or responsibility than you are ready for. Say, "I will take as much time as I need to grow."
> ▷ Give yourself permission to go at your own pace. Say, "I choose to go at my own speed regardless of what my friends are doing."
> ▷ Know that you will mature. Say, "I am maturing very well and will be able to do whatever I want in time."

▶ Special Interests

Your life as a person with ADD will be much more fulfilling if you find and develop a special interest. It may be an extracurricular activity at school or it may be entirely outside of school. You may already know what yours is. Now is the time to validate its importance for your future. If you don't have one, it's time to find yours.

Special interests are important because

they are likely to motivate you to continue your education.

they serve to focus your attention because you are doing something you like or love to do.

they act as a bright spot if you feel you live in a dull world.

they teach you that you can do something really well.

they may become the focus for a life-long interest or career.

You know something is a **special** interest because

> ▷ you love to do it.
> ▷ you do it whether you have to or not.
> ▷ you continue to engage in it over time.
> ▷ you cannot imagine life without it.

Your special interest may seem frivolous or impractical to other people but if you love it, stick with it. Some examples are

sports	bird watching	buying and selling junk
trivia	music	car racing

List your special interests here. Include those you had when you were a young child.

Name of activity	How long you've had it
_____	_____
_____	_____
_____	_____
_____	_____
_____	_____

Now, give yourself permission to continue to enjoy your special activities. It doesn't matter what other people think. If you enjoy your interest, do it.

▷ You may keep your special interest as a hobby
▷ It may lead you to career goals

When others try to tell you your interest is impractical, say,

"I appreciate your input, but I'll take responsibility for my expenses."
"I realize you are trying to help me, but I'm going to pursue my interest anyway."

To turn your interest into a career, find people who make their living doing it. Visit with them. It's all right to call ahead and ask if you can interview them. Or, if their business is open to the public, you may just drop by and strike up a conversation. Find out

▷ how the person got into the business.
▷ how training was achieved or skills were developed.
▷ what they like about being in their line of work.
▷ what the liabilities are.
▷ how they got started, financially and otherwise.
   Did someone underwrite the start-up costs?
   Did the person work two jobs?
   Does the person have a silent partner who puts up
      the money in exchange for talent?

Then, make up your own mind and take responsibility for your decision.

People to contact about your hobby or interest:

Name	Phone Number
_____	_____
_____	_____
_____	_____
_____	_____
_____	_____
_____	_____
_____	_____
_____	_____
_____	_____
_____	_____
_____	_____

► Working before Further Schooling

If you are fed up with school or are failing in school, don't know what you want to do with the rest of your life, feel you are not ready for college, or desire to see new places and have new experiences, you are a prime candidate for getting out of school for a while and trying your hand at working.

If you are still in high school but are not doing well, it may be a good idea to consider leaving school. You can take the GED test later and get your high school diploma that way. There are some implications for later entrance into a four-year institution, however. For example, some universities require thirty or more hours at a junior college or specific scores on the SAT or ACT before admission is granted. But the benefits of leaving high school may be worth these limitations.

Some people feel ready to take the GED as soon as allowed after they leave high school. Others prefer to wait several years. GED classes are held in most towns. Inquire about these through your local school system, the public library, or an information and referral service.

Next, get a job—any job—as soon as possible. The biggest danger you face is having nothing to do and no plans. You need a structure in order to move forward in the world.

Do you know how to get a job?

_____ yes _____ no

167

Can you fill out a job application neatly?

_____ yes _____ no

Do you know how to dress to go on an interview?

_____ yes _____ no

Do you know you need to call or go back to check and see how your job search is coming?

_____ yes _____ no

Do you realize that you need to keep looking until you have actually landed a job?

_____ yes _____ no

Job search pointers

1. Realize that without much education you will probably have to take a minimum-wage job at first. You can work your way up within most businesses, however.
2. Start job hunting early in the day. One exception is in businesses that are busy that time of day. Wait until a lull in their activities.
3. Dress neatly, with your shirt tucked in if you're a man and with modest, attractive clothes if you're a woman. No mini-skirts and not too much makeup.
4. Consider transportation when job hunting. You don't want to have to spend a lot of your money on getting to and from work.
5. If a business says they are not hiring, ask if you may fill out an application anyway.
6. You can usually take the applications home. If you do, keep them neat. It is best to fill them out right away so you do not get distracted and fail to finish them.
7. Do not assume that you have a job just because you turn in an application or someone says they'll let you know. Often managers don't know how to say they don't want to hire you, so they put you off. Keep looking until you are actually offered a job.
8. Try different kinds of jobs to get more experience.
9. Consider the value additional education would be in getting a job.

► Gathering Information

If you have been out of school for a while, you may want to start slowly. Consider taking one class at first. It is important to set yourself up for success. Remember, you **can** do it!

Many schools have special services for students who have been out of school for a period of time. People who have ADD are frequently able to get special help. Contact the Office of Students with Disabilities.

Write their phone number here: _____

Often special interest groups are identified in this way. For example, a women's center.

My special interest group is _____

The telephone number of my special interest group is_____

To find out what you need to return to school do the following:

1. Call the admissions office of any schools you wish to consider.

   Phone number _____

2. Ask for a catalogue. (Sometimes there is a charge of a few dollars.)
3. Look through the catalogue to see what majors fit the special interests you identified on page 166. Programs that fit your special interests are on pages

   _____, _____, and _____ of the catalogue.

4. Call the department that teaches your major and ask to talk with someone about departmental requirements (requirements to graduate with a particular major) and what you need to do in order to be successful.

   The phone number of the department is_____

   The name of the faculty member I need to speak with is _____

   Phone number _____

   Notes on what the person says _____

   _____

   _____

   _____

   _____

169

5. Consider whether you want to meet those requirements.

6. If you do not have a major in mind, talk to someone at
   the counseling center or in liberal arts about getting
   required courses out of the way. (All schools require
   everyone to take core courses. You can get these out of
   the way while you're deciding about a major.

   The counseling center number is _____

7. Register.

   My date and time of registration is _____

▶ Brokering the System

Brokering the college system means learning how to get what
you need and want from college. When you know what to do
and how to do it, you will feel much less frustrated about even
the biggest school. Your job is to learn to be efficient at using
what the college has to offer to help you overcome the effects
of your ADD.

Do one thing at a time. Check off each item as you complete it.

_____ 1. Before you go to college, be sure you have an
updated copy of the report that verifies you have
ADD.

_____ 2. Call or write to the Office of Handicapped
Student Services. (Some colleges give a different
name to this service but the registration or information people will know what you mean.)

The phone number is _____

Tell them

when you plan to enter school.
what your handicap or handicaps are.
what services you anticipate needing.

_____ 3. Talk with the person who evaluated you or draw
from your own experience about what services
would be most helpful to you. Some typical ones
are

tutoring
untimed test situations
a quiet place to take tests

being given multiple-choice tests

the ability to tape lectures

guidance in choosing classes

someone to take notes for you

someone to identify important material from
lectures and readings

support if you begin to feel overwhelmed or
have questions

a special advocate who understands ADD and
can intervene on your behalf with professors

4. If you did not meet the director of handicapped student services before getting on campus, do so immediately. Introduce yourself **before** you have any trouble.

That person's name is_____

Ask for services that will make your life easier.

Make a long-range plan whether you know your major or not. If you do not know what you want to major in, find out what services are available to help you find both what you like and what fits you.

Talk about the number and kind of classes in which you are planning to enroll for your present semester or quarter.

Find out the guidelines for dropping a class, including the date when you can withdraw without jeopardizing your grade point average.

Put that date here and on your calendar

_____

Continue to use this service throughout your college career.

Ask for whatever services you need.

Remember:

Winners make use of support services.

You are a winner!

Use this space for notes.

_____

_____

_____

_____

_____

_____

_____

_____

_____

_____

_____

_____

_____

_____

_____

_____

_____

_____

_____

_____

_____

_____

_____

_____

_____

_____

_____

_____

_____

_____

▶ The Logistics of Your Education

Dealing with the details involved in acquiring a college education can often seem more difficult than the academic work. This is true for all people, but having ADD increases the need to gain special help to organize and manage those details. It is a good idea to plan ahead so you will know what to do to handle the logistics of

1. registration   3. selection of a major   5. living arrangements
2. course load   4. dropping a course

You can avoid being penalized because you simply didn't know how or what to do. For example, too many people with ADD have severely hurt their grade point averages because they failed to properly drop a class. The following guidelines can help you avoid trouble.

▶ Schedule of Hours

For your success in college, it is important that you develop a structure that fits you. It needs to be handcrafted to fit your personal style. And, you need to remember that you can change it if you find a better way of doing things as you proceed through school. Though you may not always have the ability to get exactly what you want, do the best you can.

Consider the following:

The number of credits to take. Do not overload yourself initially. Try a maximum of fifteen credit hours. That way you can drop one class and still remain a fully enrolled student.

The types of classes to take. If you have one lab course, don't sign up for another, especially at the beginning. Balance a heavy reading class, such as humanities or English literature with one that has little reading. Try to take something in your major area so that you can feel like you are progressing in the direction you want.

The time of day for your classes to meet. If you are a morning person, you will probably do better if you sign up for classes that meet early in the day.

Make out a sample schedule for yourself on the next page after talking with an advisor. If you have a sport or group performance activity such as band, put those times in first. Then sketch in your class periods. Next, add extracurricular activities, study and mealtimes, and time for entertainment. Be sure to schedule time to watch TV if you want.

▶ Daily Activity Schedule

Name: _____ Date: _____

Description: _____

	Mon	Tues	Wed	Thurs	Fri	Sat	Sun
7:00 a.m.							
8:00 a.m.							
9:00 a.m.							
10:00 a.m.							
11:00 a.m.							
12:00 noon							
1:00 p.m.							
2:00 p.m.							
3:00 p.m.							
4:00 p.m.							
5:00 p.m.							
6:00 p.m.							
7:00 p.m.							
8:00 p.m.							
9:00 p.m.							
10:00 p.m.							
11:00 p.m.							
12:00 midnight							

▶ Choosing a Major

Choosing a major can be a frustrating experience for any college student, but when you also have ADD, it can become overwhelming. ADD students become easily bored when locked into one subject, but are also overwhelmed by too many choices. Most college counseling offices offer free career testing to students. You can get help there.

Earlier you took into account your special interests when considering a major. Now, it is time to go further.

Ask yourself the following:

1. What are my academic strengths? _____

_____

2. What are my academic weaknesses? _____

_____

3. What am I interested in doing for a living? _____

_____

4. How hard do I want to work in college? _____

5. How long will it take me to complete this major? _____ years (Give yourself permission to take five years or more to finish.)

6. Do I have outside interests that will take my time? _____

List them _____

_____

7. Now that I've focused on a major area of interest, how can I make use of what I learn in the work-a-day world? _____

_____

8. Will I need to go to graduate school in order to get a job in the field of my study. Is there a faculty member with whom I can talk?

Name _____ Telephone _____

Is there an advanced student with whom I can talk?

Name _____ Telephone _____

Now, select one or two possible majors. Begin to take courses in these areas a little at a time and see how you feel about the subject. You may try to get a summer job in a related area. Consider volunteering a few hours a week in the area of your major to see if you like being involved in the job.

▶ Dropping a Class

If you misjudge the amount of work needed for a particular class, or you get a professor who is especially hard for you to understand, you may want to drop a class. Here are some guidelines. Consider the following:

1. Do I really want to drop it?
2. Have I been working smart?
3. Have I been using the services of the Office of the Handicapped to see whether I can get some help?
4. Have I been goofing off and just need to buckle down?

Always talk over any problem you are having in a class with the professor, graduate teaching assistant, or counselor. There may be help available that you don't know about. If you decide you've done all you can do and you are still in over your head, drop the course. **But,** be sure to actually drop it in time. Check your catalogue and see how late in the semester or quarter you can drop a course before you must take an F.

Fill in the following:

At my school, I must drop a course by the _____ week

of the semester or quarter. I will lose _____ dollars.

If someone other than yourself is paying for your schooling, let that person know what you are doing and why. Be honest with yourself and others.

If you have only gotten behind in a class, most universities will allow you to take an incomplete so that you can finish a paper after the semester is over. Ask your professor.

▶ Living Arrangements

There are several different kinds of living arrangements for students at college. Your choice will depend on several conditions: your age, marital status, finances, and personal preferences. Your options include living in a dorm, off-campus, and at home.

> ▷ Dorm life
> Pros
> Few responsibilities
> Other students to help you out with questions
> Peer support (good if others are studying)
> Social life

Cons

Often noisy

Lots of partying

Overstimulating

▷ Off-campus (getting your own apartment)

Pros

May be quieter

Amount of partying is up to you

Less stimulating

More privacy

Cons

More responsibility

Lack of peer support

▷ At home (If you are married, this is probably essential.)

Pros

Support (you hope) from family members

Good, home-cooked meals

Less responsibility (If you live with parents)

Firm limits that help you stay on task

Cons

Study groups may be harder to come by

Parents may try to control your studying or activities

Can be hard on your family if you are working and going to school, and so don't have time for them

▶ Coping with Poor Teaching

Let's suppose you have done all the things recommended in this section. You are in control of yourself and your ADD. But you encounter a poor teacher—someone who does not know how to teach or has poor interpersonal skills. What can you do?

First, assess the situation by answering the following questions. This will help you define the problem.

1. Does the teacher explain the material in different ways?
2. Is the teacher open to questions about the teaching?
3. Does the teacher clearly state what is expected to get a particular grade?
4. Are the exams stated in the same terms in which the material is taught?
5. Does the teacher allow enough time for you to take your exams?
6. Can you tell what is expected of you?
7. Is the teacher poorly prepared?

All of these questions are about the way the material is taught and tested. Wherever you have "no" answers, you can expect to experience difficulty with the material.

The following questions relate to the teacher's manner of interaction and behavior.

1. Is there a supportive atmosphere in the classroom that lets you know the teacher is behind you—on your team?
2. Does the teacher take the time to get to know the students?
3. Does the teacher verbally abuse or embarrass students?
4. Does the teacher use a scolding tone with students?
5. Does the teacher seem absentminded?
6. Is the teacher impatient?
7. Does the teacher use class time to talk about himself or his pet subjects more than about the concepts or material?
8. Does the teacher appear anxious, depressed, or distraught?
9. Is the teacher overly critical or a perfectionist?

These questions are intended to describe the teacher's approach to other people as well as feelings about herself.

Fill in the following:

My teacher, named _____

does the following things that I dislike.

_____

_____

_____

_____

_____

My teacher acts in the following way that I dislike:

_____

_____

_____

_____

_____

When you feel upset about a teacher, it is more difficult to do the classwork. Be aware of your feelings. Are you so angry in class that all you think about during the lecture is how awful the teacher is? This will tend to distract you. Or you may have an angry look on your face, causing the teacher not to like you. Remember, teachers are people, too. You earn your grades by your own work, but alienating the teacher could possibly hurt your grade. And it will certainly hurt your ability to get the extra help and explanations you need. It's really no different than working to get along with coworkers or bosses—your life will be easier if you learn to be tolerant.

To help you out, I ask you to write down your dislikes. Once they are on paper, you can begin to plan more clearly what you want to do about your situation.

▷ **Step 1:** Vent your emotions

People with ADD often feel better if they are simply able to complain about someone or something that is bothersome.

Find someone who is a good listener and tell the person it is not necessary to respond to this complaining.

In your complaining, you can *blame* the teacher for getting bad grades, question his character, or basically describe how unfair the situation is. (For people who do not have ADD, it is often hard to hear this biased kind of monologue. They often want to try to *reason* with the person with ADD. Explain to them that you really just need to complain and that you will take action to improve the situation once you have vented your feelings.)

Vent your feelings for five minutes. In that time you can get them all out. Then release your angry attachment to them and get ready to go on to more constructive ways to handle your situation.

From here on out, no more complaining.

▷ **Step 2:** Make a plan to improve the situation.

If the problem is with the teacher's behavior, ask for help from someone other than another person who is also angry about the teacher. Figure out together *what* the teacher needs. You can do this by carefully observing the teacher.

▷ What motivates the teacher?
▷ Does the teacher like to be in control?
▷ Does the teacher seem insecure?
▷ What kind of students does the teacher seem to like?
▷ How can I get along better with the teacher? (You don't have to *like* the teacher to do this.)

179

Make a plan to get the teacher on your side—to like you.

- ▷ If the teacher is motivated by status, tell him how you respect teachers. If the teacher is motivated by dialoguing with students who ask a lot of questions, then you ask a lot of questions.
- ▷ With a controlling teacher, act humble or at least be quiet and non-confrontive. (Hard for a lot of people with ADD, I know, but do it anyway.)
- ▷ Act supportive of an insecure teacher saying, "I really appreciate the way you have been helping me. Thank you."
- ▷ Mimic the behavior of students the teacher likes.
- ▷ Show interest in the subject and the teacher's approach.

If the teacher is nice enough but doesn't know how to teach

- ▷ get in a study group to learn outside of class.
- ▷ learn on your own if you are a good reader.
- ▷ get a student who is majoring in the subject to act as a teacher—say what your problem is in the class and that you need an outside teacher.

Know that you are in class for one reason—to learn as much and get as good a grade as you possibly can. Remember, you do not need to *prove* you are *right* or that the teacher is *wrong*.

Write your plan of attack below.

_____

_____

_____

_____

_____

_____

_____

_____

_____

_____

_____

Your education is your responsibility and you want to take control of it, not be a passive victim. Ultimately, you may decide to drop the class because the teacher is so bad. But *you* will have made the decision. You *can* succeed in school, despite these obstacles.

► Don't Fool Yourself

Going to school is hard work. Even if you have a light load initially, you will have to develop self-discipline to be successful at school. Below are some guidelines to help you keep on track and not fool yourself.

Ask yourself weekly the following:

1. Am I failing to keep up with class?

_____ yes _____ no

2. Am I tending to put off writing papers or doing research?

_____ yes _____ no

3. Am I spending a lot of time with my girl (boy) friend?

_____ yes _____ no

4. If "yes" to 3, are we studying together?

_____ yes _____ no

5. Do I drink a lot?

_____ yes _____ no

6. Am I using drugs or experimenting with them?

_____ yes _____ no

7. Am I skipping class?

_____ yes _____ no

8. Do I stay up so late that I can't get up in the morning?

_____ yes _____ no

9. Do I isolate myself from others or feel down?

_____ yes _____ no

10. If I'm honest with myself, am I worried I might fail?

_____ yes _____ no

11. Would I rather be working than be in school?

_____ yes _____ no

12. Am I putting off dropping a class or classes?

_____ yes _____ no

13. Have I put off telling my parents or spouse that I am not making the grade?

_____ yes _____ no

14. Do I feel guilty about the way I'm handling college?

_____ yes _____ no

15. Do I feel that most of my professors don't know what they are doing?

_____ yes _____ no

The more "yes" answers you have, the greater the danger that you are setting yourself up for failure. You don't deserve that. You can be a winner.

Most of the situations are ones that you can do something about. But you must be honest. Rather than blaming your poor grades on someone else, take responsibility to do something about your situation.

▷ Talk with your professor.
▷ Go to the handicapped student office for help.
▷ Go to the counseling center for assistance.
▷ Talk with your dorm graduate assistant.
▷ Let your parents (spouse) know you are having trouble.
▷ Let any of the above people help you figure out why you are having trouble. Then, construct a new plan for success.

Give yourself permission to drop out of school if you feel overwhelmed. Work for a while. Remember, maturity lags for people who have ADD. You will be surprised how smart you can become as you gain practical experience. Also know that college is not for everyone. You **can** be successful without it. Do your best at whatever you love and know you will come out a winner.

INDEX